IMPROVE YOUR VISION

VISION

Without Glasses or Contact Lenses

The AVI Program

Dr. Steven M. Beresford,
Dr. David W. Muris, Dr. Merrill J. Allen,
Dr. Francis A. Young

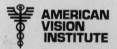

AMERICAN
VISION
INSTITUTE

A FIRESIDE BOOK
Published by Simon & Schuster

FIRESIDE
Rockefeller Center
1230 Avenue of the Americas
New York, NY 10020

Copyright © 1996 by Dr. Steven M. Beresford

FIRESIDE and colophon are registered trademarks
of Simon & Schuster Inc.

Designed by Irving Perkins Associates, Inc.

Manufactured in the United States of America

11 13 15 17 19 20 18 16 14 12

Library of Congress Cataloging-in-Publication Data
Improve your vision without glasses or contact lenses : the AVI
program / Steven M. Beresford . . . [et al.].
        p.   cm.
1. Visual training.   I. Beresford, Steven M.
        RE960.I47   1996
617.7—dc20   96-22038
                                                    CIP

ISBN 0-684-81438-2

NOTICE TO ALL READERS

This book is an educational tool that can teach you how to see more clearly, comfortably, and efficiently. It is not intended to be a medical or assistive device, nor is it a substitute for diagnosis or treatment by an optometrist or ophthalmologist. The techniques presented here are considered to be completely safe, but should not be used without first consulting an optometrist or ophthalmologist to determine if any disease or other disorder requiring specialized treatment is present.

CONTENTS

1

HOW YOUR EYES WORK

WELCOME TO THE AVI PROGRAM

The American Vision Institute (AVI) is a research organization established in 1979 that has helped pioneer some of the recent advances in
eye care. What you're about to read will probably contradict much of
what your eye doctor told you about your eyes and the way they should
be treated. However, our goal is not to discredit the eye care profession
but to improve the quality of eye care offered to the public. Pretending
that the traditional use of "corrective" lenses is safe and effective is no
longer acceptable. The public must be told the truth and given accurate
information about the alternative methods of treatment now available.
Before proceeding we'd like to briefly introduce ourselves:

- **Professor Merrill J. Allen:** Graduate of Ohio State University and
  Professor Emeritus of Optometry at Indiana University. As recip-
  ient of twenty-one professional honors including the American
  Optometric Association's Apollo Award and the British Optical
  Association's Research Medal, Professor Allen is one of the most
  highly credentialed optometrists in the United States.

- **Dr. Steven M. Beresford:** Graduate of Leicester University (UK)
  and President of the American Vision Institute. In addition to
  vision research, Dr. Beresford is an authority on nuclear chemistry
  and has published his work in major scientific journals.

- **Dr. David W. Muris:** Graduate of Southern California College of Optometry and Director of Sacramento Visioncare Optometric Center. Dr. Muris is former President of the Sacramento Valley Optometric Association, Chairman of the Yolo County Health Plan, and Regional Chairman of the Optometric Extension Program.

- **Professor Francis A. Young:** Graduate of Ohio State University and Professor Emeritus of Psychology at Washington State University. As the recipient of eleven professional honors, including the American Optometric Association's Apollo Award, Professor Young is one of the world's leading authorities on myopia.

This book, the AVI Program, is written for busy people who want hard facts and fast results. So we're not going to waste your valuable time with long-winded introductions, prefaces, or forewords. Instead, we're going to teach you some important techniques that you can start practicing right away. Most of what you're about to read will be unfamiliar to you, so don't panic if you don't totally understand everything immediately. It's really quite simple once you get used to the new words and concepts. *You should approach the AVI Program as a course of study. We suggest you read each chapter three times and everything will soon sink in and become perfectly clear.*

The most important purpose of the AVI Program is to help you achieve a significant improvement in your vision within one month. Our basic premise is that you should actively care for your eyes by exercising them regularly and developing good visual habits. This is completely different from the traditional concept of eye care, in which patients passively rely on doctors to provide progressively stronger "corrective" lenses, check for eye diseases, prescribe drugs, and perform surgery. In other words, the goal of traditional eye care is to treat the symptoms, whereas the goal of the AVI Program is to improve and possibly eliminate the underlying problem.

Like most people with poor eyesight, you've probably been told that your condition is hopeless, that you're a victim of heredity or the aging process, and that there's nothing you can do except resign yourself to stronger prescriptions and the risk of cataracts or other eye diseases as you grow older. Fortunately, there's a better way. The AVI Program will teach you some simple techniques that will empower you to actively participate in your eye care.

YOUR EYES MUST LAST A LIFETIME

Compare traditional eye care with dental care. Imagine the mess your teeth would be in if you didn't bother to clean them every day! Imagine what would happen if your dentist told you that nothing could be done except to put in bigger fillings year after year until your teeth were ruined! Now compare traditional eye care with hair care. Imagine the mess your hair would be in if you never brushed it, but merely relied on your hairdresser to cut it from time to time!

Make no mistake. Your eyes are much more important than your teeth or your hair. If you lose your teeth, you can get dentures. If you lose your hair, you can get a wig. But your eyes must last your entire lifetime. You can't replace them at any price. If you just rely on your eye doctor to prescribe stronger "corrective" lenses every few years, you aren't giving your eyes the special care and attention they deserve. Your eyes are priceless, and you should develop the habit of exercising them on a daily basis so that they become strong and healthy. You wouldn't dream of ignoring your teeth or hair, so don't ignore your eyes. It's easy to look after them properly, once you know how.

THE EYE'S BASIC STRUCTURE

The eye is an approximately spherical bag of living cells 1 inch across, filled with transparent jelly and a pressurized liquid that keeps it inflated like a balloon. At the front of the eye is the cornea, which is a window of transparent cells that allows light to enter. Just behind the cornea is the iris, which is an opaque diaphragm of colored muscle that regulates the amount of light entering the eye. The pupil is the dark hole

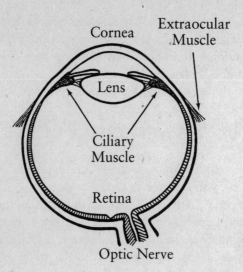

in the center of the iris, which becomes larger or smaller as the iris expands or contracts.

Immediately behind the iris is the inner lens, which is a transparent capsule of cells with the consistency of rubber that focuses light onto the retina at the back of the eye. Although the eye is usually compared to a film camera, a television camera is a better analogy because the retina is composed of specialized cells that convert light into the electrical impulses that travel up the optic nerve to the brain. Every 1/40 of a second, the retina can transmit a new image consisting of more than 100 million bits of information.

Until recently, it was thought that visual perception took place only in the brain. It is now known that the retina, which is a complex and highly organized network of nerve cells, processes the raw image for basic information such as outlines, colors, and motion. The brain completes the processing and derives more information about detail, distance, and dimension. It adds meaning and integrates the data into what you actually see. It's worth noting that the retina seems to possess a rudimentary form of intelligence and many scientists now regard it as an extension of the brain.

HOW THE EYE CHANGES FOCUS

The eye's optical system consists of two major components: the cornea and the inner lens. The cornea has almost three times as much refractive power as the inner lens. Light first passes through the cornea, which partially focuses it, then passes through the inner lens, which completes the focusing onto the retina and can adjust the focus as needed.

The eye changes focus between objects at different distances by the action of the ciliary muscle on the inner lens, thereby adjusting its shape and refractive power. It has also been theorized that the extraocular muscles can respond to emotional stress by changing the length of the eyeball and may play a minor role in the focusing process.

The ciliary muscle, a circular muscle similar to the iris, is attached to the inner lens through a microscopic meshwork of fibrous filaments known as the *zonule of Zinn*. When the ciliary muscle expands, it makes the inner lens thinner and reduces its refractive power so that far objects are focused onto the retina. When the ciliary muscle contracts, it makes the inner lens thicker and increases its refractive power so that near objects are focused onto the retina.

VISION IS TEAMWORK

Six extraocular muscles surround each eyeball and move the eyes so that they point at the same object at the same time. The power and precision required is truly amazing. During the course of a rapid eye movement lasting about 1/10 of a second, the eyeball accelerates at a tremendous rate and decelerates almost instantly. To generate enough power to do this, the extraocular muscles are approximately 200 times stronger than would be needed just to slowly turn the eyes in their sockets.

The eyes are constantly looking from object to object, detail to detail, as they scan the world and gather information. For example, as you read these words, your eyes are automatically jumping from one group of letters to the next. These jumping movements are known as *saccades*. When the eyes follow a moving object, they make a different type of movement known as *pursuits*, which are smooth and continuous. Finally, there's another type of movement known as *slow drifting*. If you stare at a small dot for more than a few seconds, your gaze will periodically drift away, then return to the dot.

In normal healthy eyes, the ciliary and extraocular muscles work together as a team, constantly adjusting to the world around us. The brain is in complete control and makes the eyes point and focus on the same object at the same time as they constantly search for new objects of interest. If the ciliary muscle malfunctions, the eyes go out of focus. If the extraocular muscles malfunction, the eyes may point at different objects. This is usually experienced as double vision, headaches, eyestrain, suppressed vision, slow reading, poor depth perception, or a tendency to bump into things.

Because the eyes are a few inches apart, each eye receives a slightly different image, like two separate cameras. The brain fuses these images together to form a three-dimensional representation of the world. Since the image in each eye is only two-dimensional, the three-dimensional image we see is really an illusion, although it is totally convincing.

WINDOWS OF THE SOUL

With their enchanting beauty and sex appeal, the eyes are like a delicate exotic flower reaching for the light. Much of this beauty is due to the iris. Quick to protect the retina from glare, the iris can contract the pupil to the size of a pinhead. In the dark, however, the iris can expand the pupil up to ⅓ inch to welcome any available light.

Although the iris automatically responds to light, it is also a sensitive barometer of emotion. Anger, fear, pleasure, and lust can all be read in the movement of the iris and the size of the pupil. Negative emotions make the pupil contract, as if to shut out the offending object. Likewise, an expanding pupil registers hidden attraction, as the eye opens up to feast on light from the object of desire.

Eyelids enhance the beauty of the eyes but have a more important biological function. By blinking every few seconds, they bathe and polish the cornea with antiseptic tears, protecting it against dryness, pollution, bacteria, and foreign objects. When a particle of dust hits the eye, it triggers a flood of tears that wash it out. Intense emotions can also bring about this natural purge. In fact, research studies suggest that the brain can use tear fluid to eliminate stress-induced toxins.

Quick to capture the light of the world, the eyes are also a mirror of the mind. Not only does the iris quickly betray hidden feelings, but eyelids, eyebrows, and eye movements are frequently used as a subtle means of communication. Because of their remarkable versatility, Saint Jerome once wrote that *"Eyes without speaking confess the secrets of the heart."*

Our language is replete with expressions such as: *"blind with rage"* or *"starry eyed"* or *"his eyes narrowed as he reached for his gun"* or *"she flashed her eyes at him"* or *"she gave him the evil eye."* In fact, eye contact is an important part of body language. Good eye contact is essential to bonding, whereas a refusal to look someone in the eye is usually a sign of guilt or fear. A hostile glare can quickly intimidate, but tearful eyes can plead for mercy with silent eloquence.

Just as emotions rise readily from the eye's lucid depths, so do reflections of the general state of health. Signs of bodily diseases, toxic substances, and dietary deficiencies often first appear in the eyes. With a careful eye examination, a skilled eye doctor can often learn of these problems long before they make their appearance elsewhere in the body. Some doctors also use a technique known as *iridology,* which is based on irregularities in the markings of the iris. These irregularities are thought to indicate diseases and other health problems.

NOW FOR SOME BASIC TERMS

Although we've tried to avoid using a lot of technical jargon, you need to know some basic terms. Please read this list a few times until you're familiar with the words and concepts. We'll explain things in more detail later.

ACCOMMODATION: The ability to change focus.

ACUITY: Clarity of vision expressed as a fraction, such as 20/150. The smaller the denominator, the better the acuity. Far acuity is usually measured at 20 feet and near acuity at 14 inches. Normal vision without "corrective" lenses is defined as 20/20 at far and 14/14 at near.

AMBLYOPIA (LAZY EYE): A condition in which the brain suppresses the nerve impulses from one eye, giving it subnormal acuity. In most cases, there is nothing basically wrong with the suppressed eye, although it may turn inward or outward. A person with amblyopia is known as an *amblyope*. (PRONOUNCED AMBLEE-OPIA)

ASTIGMATISM: A visual problem in which the eyeball and/or cornea is warped. The result is uneven focusing of light on the retina so that the image is blurred and distorted. Astigmatism usually diminishes acuity at all distances.

CATARACT: A degenerative eye disease in which cells inside the eye's inner lens die and obstruct the passage of light. A cataract is not a tumor or growth but simply the accumulation of dead cells, which makes the inner lens cloudy. Cataracts can be removed surgically but complications from surgery sometimes cause blindness.

CILIARY MUSCLE: The circular muscle that surrounds the inner lens and makes it change shape.

CONVERGENCE: The ability to point the eyes at the same object at the same time.

"CORRECTIVE" LENSES: Glasses or contact lenses that treat the symptoms of poor vision by compensating for the eye's optical defects.

"Corrective" lenses, also known as "compensatory" lenses, don't actually correct the underlying visual problem but only modify the light before it enters the eye.

DEVELOPMENTAL VISUAL PROBLEMS: Problems arising when a child's visual system fails to develop properly. Developmental visual problems can remain undetected throughout the person's entire lifetime.

DIOPTER: The unit of measurement of the refractive power of a lens, equal to the reciprocal of the focal length in meters. For example, a lens with a focal length of ⅓ meters has 3 diopters (+3.00D) of refractive power. The stronger the lens, the more diopters.

DRY EYE SYNDROME: A condition in which the tear glands don't function properly, producing insufficient tear fluid or tear fluid with the wrong composition.

ENVIRONMENTAL THEORY: The theory that environmental factors such as stress, lighting, nutrition, posture, and excessive close work are the major causes of visual problems such as eyestrain, astigmatism, myopia, and cataract.

EXTRAOCULAR MUSCLES: A group of six muscles that surround the eyeball and move it in different directions.

GENETIC THEORY: The theory that visual problems are genetically determined.

GLAUCOMA: A degenerative eye disease usually caused by blockages in the eye's drainage system that increase the pressure inside the eyeball. Glaucoma often damages the optic nerve and is officially listed as a major cause of blindness.

HYPEROPIA (FARSIGHTEDNESS): A visual problem in which the person sees far objects better than near objects. A person with hyperopia is called a *hyperope*. (PRONOUNCED HYPER-OH-PIA)

IATROGENIC PROBLEMS: Secondary problems caused by the treatment itself, such as side effects caused by drugs, complications caused by surgery, or loss of natural focusing power caused by "corrective" lenses. (PRONOUNCED YATRA-GENIC)

LASER SURGERY: The use of a laser to destroy cellular tissue, for example, treating glaucoma by drilling tiny drainage holes in the eye. Lasers are also used to treat myopia and astigmatism by vaporizing part of the cornea, thereby changing its curvature and refractive power.

MACULAR DEGENERATION: A degenerative eye disease in which cells die in the central part of the retina at the back of the eye, resulting in partial blindness.

MINUS LENS: A lens that makes objects appear smaller. Minus lenses have negative diopters of refractive power, for example, −5.00D, and are used to treat myopia.

MYOPIA (NEARSIGHTEDNESS): A visual problem in which the person sees near objects better than far objects. A person with myopia is called a *myope*. (PRONOUNCED MY-OPIA)

MYOPIA MORBIDITY: Degenerative eye diseases caused by or associated with myopia, including cataract, glaucoma, macular degeneration, and retinal detachment. Myopia is officially listed as a major cause of blindness.

NEARPOINT STRESS: The major visual stress factor, caused by too much reading, computers, TV, or other close work.

OPHTHALMOLOGIST: A doctor who treats eye diseases by means of drugs and surgery. Many ophthalmologists also treat visual problems by means of "corrective" lenses or refractive surgery.

OPTICIAN: A technician who dispenses glasses and contact lenses.

OPTOMETRIST: A traditional optometrist is a doctor who treats visual problems by means of "corrective" lenses. A behavioral optometrist is a doctor who treats visual problems by means of vision therapy. Most optometrists are also licensed to prescribe various drugs and perform minor surgery.

ORTHOKERATOLOGY: A procedure that changes the curvature and refractive power of the cornea by means of special contact lenses.

PLUS LENS: A lens that makes objects appear to be larger. Plus lenses have positive diopters of refractive power, for example, +5.00D, and are used to treat presbyopia and hyperopia.

PRESBYOPIA (AGING EYES): A visual problem in which the eye loses its focusing power due to the aging process, especially in people over forty. If the person previously had good vision, near objects may become blurred although distant objects can usually be seen clearly. If the person previously had myopia, astigmatism, or hyperopia, bifocals are usually prescribed. A person with presbyopia is called a *presbyope.* (PRONOUNCED PRESBEE-OPIA)

PROGRESSIVE UNDERCORRECTION: The use of a series of progressively weaker "corrective" lenses to improve vision and increase the eye's natural focusing power, usually in conjunction with vision therapy.

REFRACTIVE ERROR: A measurement of the eye's inability to focus light from a distant object onto the retina. Refractive errors are measured in terms of power of the "corrective" lens needed to compensate for them. For example, a −5.00D myope has 5 diopters of myopia, whereas a +3.00D hyperope has 3 diopters of hyperopia.

REFRACTIVE POWER: The ability of a lens to focus light. The lens can be an external lens or one of the eye's optical components such as the cornea.

RETINAL DETACHMENT: A leading cause of blindness in which the retina detaches from the supporting tissue at the back of the eyeball.

RK SURGERY: The use of a scalpel to make radial cuts in the cornea, thereby changing its curvature and refractive power.

STRABISMUS (CROSSED EYES): A condition in which the eyes point in different directions, causing double vision or suppressed vision in one eye.

STRESS-RELIEVING GLASSES: Special glasses that improve the performance of the visual system, usually in conjunction with vision therapy.

VISION: The total awareness resulting from information obtained by the eyes. Vision also depends on past experiences, current emotions, expectations, stress, nutrition, the general state of health, posture, bodily activities, and information received from the other senses.

VISION THERAPY: Commonly known as *eye exercises*, vision therapy consists of various techniques that improve the performance of the eyes and visual system, including acupressure, stress reduction, behavior modification, biofeedback, hydrotherapy, hypnosis, nutrition, ocular calisthenics, yoga, and syntonics. If lenses or prisms are used, vision therapy is referred to as *optometric visual training*.

COMMON VISUAL PROBLEMS

VISION DOMINATES YOUR LIFE

Basic vision is a six-step process that usually takes less than a second from start to finish:

1. The brain observes the world using peripheral vision, sees an object of interest, and decides to gather information about the object. At this stage the eyes are not pointing directly at the object.

2. The brain then determines the relative position of the object and computes the trajectory and power needed to move the eyes to point directly at it.

3. The brain then directs the extraocular muscles to move the eyes so that they point directly at the object.

4. The brain then directs each ciliary muscle to focus its lens and make the object clearer.

5. The brain then gathers information about the object and determines its significance.

6. Finally, the brain decides whether or not to respond to the object and uses the eyes to coordinate whatever bodily movements are needed.

VISION IS LEARNED

The mystery of vision has intrigued philosophers, doctors, and scientists for centuries. More than 2,000 years ago the Greek doctor Alcmaeon discovered that the eyes are connected to the brain. He correctly theorized that visual sensations come together in the brain and are then integrated with memory and thought. Although major advances were made in the anatomy of the eye during the nineteenth century, it was not until the 1930s that optometrists, psychologists, and educators discovered that vision is learned.

This discovery came as a big surprise because it was previously thought that vision was automatic, like breathing or digestion. Studies of child development showed this to be incorrect. Although we are born with basic visual reflexes, we learn how to use our eyes. Just opening the eyes doesn't automatically generate a coherent picture, like switching on a TV set. In fact, vision is a learned set of more than twenty separate skills.

In addition to forming images, the visual system is involved in the ability to determine the size, speed, distance, and position of an object; the ability to estimate the composition, texture, weight, purpose, and age of an object without touching it; the ability to compare one object with another; the ability to maintain balance, posture, and direction; and the ability to read and interpret written words, signs, and symbols. These skills are learned and refined throughout childhood and remain fairly constant throughout most of adult life until they decline in old age. Some children learn them quickly and easily. Others develop defective visual skills that can seriously hinder their progress and prevent them from doing well at school or in the workplace, resulting in a lifetime of underachievement.

This is how the learning process takes place. Immediately after being born, babies see the world but don't understand what they're looking at. They find themselves in a strange continuum of meaningless shapes and bright colors. Nevertheless, they can focus and coordinate their eyes to some extent almost immediately. As time goes by, their sense of touch makes them aware of their body, and they learn that some of the new shapes and colors belong to it. They also learn that many other shapes and colors belong to things that are not their body. As they come into contact with different objects, they gradually differentiate themselves from the rest of the world and establish a separate identity. Their sense of self and understanding of reality gradually emerge as they learn how to use their eyes and interpret the information gathered by them.

THREE SURPRISING CONCLUSIONS

The fact that vision is learned leads to some fascinating and quite unexpected conclusions. First, the amount of learning, and hence the development of the visual system, depends on the experiences of the person. For example, children raised in bright, colorful homes with lots of different stimuli usually have better visual systems than children raised in dark, dingy squalor. The influence of the environment is enormous, even with adults. Many people who work under fluorescent lights develop visual problems. So do many people who spend long hours at computers.

Second, each person has a different way of seeing, known as a *visual style,* which depends on how that person learned to operate his or her eyes and visual system. Just as you have your own unique way of walking and talking, so you see the world in your own unique way. Some people develop good visual skills quickly and easily during their formative years. Others fail to do this and spend their lives handicapped by inferior vision. Many people develop good visual skills as children that are damaged later in life through stress, poor nutrition, or the aging process. The perception of space also varies widely. Some people see the world as completely flat; others see it in three dimensions. Many people are trapped in a bubble of clarity only a few inches across; others can see stars but can't read up close.

Third, like any other learned skill, vision can be improved by practice. This vitally important fact forms the foundation of vision therapy. The amount of improvement can be substantial. After treating almost 10,000 patients with the techniques in this book, it is our professional opinion that no matter how bad a person's eyesight, vision therapy can improve it. There is no doubt that the visual system responds to therapy, often with dramatic results. You should not limit yourself by thinking that you're too old or that your vision is too bad. The visual system is suprisingly flexible and older people often get better results than younger people.

THE MYTH OF 20/20 VISION

Most people, including the majority of eye doctors, confuse eyesight with vision. Strictly speaking, *eyesight* refers to the perception of the retinal image, whereas *vision* refers to the many different ways the brain processes that image. To avoid getting bogged down in technical jargon, we'll also use eyesight and vision interchangeably, even though they are rather different. However, there's one important difference that you should know about. Like most people, you probably believe that 20/20 is perfect vision. In fact, this is an older point of view that is only partly true, dating back to the time when the eye care profession was in its infancy.

The first eyechart was developed in the middle of the nineteenth century by Hermann Snellen, an ophthalmologist who used different sized letters to measure blurred vision at a distance. The Snellen chart is the one with the big E at the top and smaller letters below that you see in most doctors' offices. Although the Snellen chart is a valuable diagnostic tool, it measures only one visual skill, far acuity, which is not always the most important one.

When the other visual skills are not up to par, problems often arise that can be just as serious as blurred distance vision. Unfortunately, when children learn how to see, there is a major drawback. They don't get feedback from parents or teachers unless something is obviously wrong, such as a lazy eye or crossed eyes. If the eyes appear to be normal, there's no way of telling just by looking at them if the visual system is developing properly.

DEVELOPMENTAL VISUAL PROBLEMS

When a child mispronounces a word, the parent or teacher notices the error and corrects it. In this way, the child receives feedback and learns how to speak properly. However, when a child learns how to use his or her eyes, it's almost impossible for the parent or teacher to know if the process is proceeding smoothly. Nature doesn't automatically produce efficient visual systems.

Many children have perfect 20/20 vision but are burdened with a host of hidden visual problems. Unless steps are taken to detect and correct these problems, they usually continue unnoticed throughout the person's lifetime, causing endless frustration, failure, and underachievement. These problems are called *developmental visual problems* and can also be superimposed on other visual problems, such as myopia or presbyopia.

Because most developmental visual problems exist below the surface, they prevent the visual system from functioning smoothly and can seriously affect a person's life without his or her realizing it. For example, people with poor eye movements usually have difficulty reading or adding up numbers and are less likely to succeed in the workplace. Likewise, people with a lazy eye or poor peripheral vision are more likely to bump into things and have accidents.

Fortunately, vision therapy can usually correct these problems by making the visual system more efficient and more balanced. In many cases, the result is faster reading, fewer errors, and better comprehension. Once the blockages are removed, the intellect may blossom. In fact, in some cases the person's IQ increased by fifteen points after vision therapy, simply because the brain was no longer burdened by an inefficient visual system.

HOW TO DETECT DEVELOPMENTAL VISUAL PROBLEMS

A standard eye examination by a traditional eye doctor can't detect developmental visual problems. Only behavioral optometrists are fully equipped to evaluate the inner workings of the visual system. However, the following checklist will enable you to determine if you have any of the more common developmental visual problems:

1. Can you cross your eyes and see both sides of your nose at the same time?   Yes ☐   No ☐

2. Can you look at something 3 inches away without seeing a double image?   Yes ☐   No ☐

3. Do you get frequent headaches from reading or using a computer?   Yes ☐   No ☐

4. Does one of your eyes drift inward or outward when you are very tired?   Yes ☐   No ☐

5. Are you a slow reader and often lose your place or have to reread things?   Yes ☐   No ☐

6. Do you suffer from motion sickness or vertigo?   Yes ☐   No ☐

7. Are you clumsy and often bump into things or can't tell left from right?   Yes ☐   No ☐

If you answered *no* to items 1 or 2, or *yes* to any of the other questions, you probably have a developmental visual problem. Although the AVI Program will help in many cases, if the problem persists you should consider doing extra vision therapy under the care of a behavioral optometrist.

HOW TO DETECT A LAZY EYE

Most people have a dominant eye and a weaker eye, just like being left-handed or right-handed. This is normal as long as the weaker eye isn't too badly suppressed. Here are two simple tests to help you find out:

1. Make a large dot on a blank wall and sit about 10 feet in front of it. Hold the index finger of your dominant hand 6 inches in front of you and look at the dot on the wall in line with the finger. Hold your hand so that you can see two finger images with your peripheral vision, one on either side of the dot. The left finger image corresponds to the right eye and the right finger image corresponds to the left eye. While looking directly at the dot, notice if one of the two finger images is fainter or more transparent than the other. If so, that finger image corresponds to your weaker eye. If it's considerably fainter than the other finger image, you're probably suppressing the image and have a lazy eye.

2. Continue to look at the dot and touch your chin with your index finger. Now quickly stretch out your hand to arm's length and point directly at the dot. As before, you should see two finger images. You should notice that the finger image from your dominant eye is doing the pointing and the other finger image is off to one side. Repeat the test with the index finger of your other hand.

Now make a note of the results of the two tests:

Right eye:	Dominant ☐	Weaker ☐	Lazy ☐
Left eye:	Dominant ☐	Weaker ☐	Lazy ☐

WHY GOOD VISION GOES BAD

Traditional eye care is based on the unproven theory that common visual problems such as myopia, hyperopia, astigmatism, and even strabismus are the result of genetically deformed eyeballs. According to this theory, visual problems are the result of genetic defects and therefore can't be prevented or cured. Even presbyopia and cataracts are considered to be genetically determined. Although the evidence to the contrary is overwhelming, the genetic theory of poor vision is still taught at most optometric colleges and medical schools. We'll explain why later.

The truth is that human beings evolved to have excellent vision, especially at a distance, because our ancestors were hunters and warriors whose survival depended on it. People with defective vision couldn't hunt successfully or were killed by enemies or predators, so they didn't survive. Dead men don't tell tales. Neither do they reproduce. The fact that humans beings survived and prospered means that we too have the potential for good vision as an essential component of our genetic heritage.

In fact, almost everyone is born with normal healthy eyes and less than 2 percent of children have deformed eyeballs. As further proof that our ancestors were hunters and warriors, almost all children have a small amount of hyperopia. This is biological "insurance" that enables the person to see enemies or predators far away, even if the eyeballs are not completely perfect.

Dramatic proof that poor vision is usually not inherited came from investigations of preindustrial societies such as North American Indians and Polynesian Islanders. Almost everyone in these societies except presbyopes had excellent vision and myopia was practically nonexistent. The most important of these investigations was carried out in 1968 by AVI's Professor Young, who led a research team to Alaska to study Eskimo families in the process of being assimilated into the American mainstream. This provided a splendid opportunity to test the genetic theory because the parents were illiterate, whereas their children were the first generation to go through school. According to the genetic theory, the parents' and children's visual systems should have been almost identical, with little or no myopia.

What Young discovered stunned the eye care profession. Of 130 parents, 128 had excellent distance vision and only 2 had myopia. This was expected because the tribe was living the typical Eskimo lifestyle of hunting and fishing. One parent had 0.25D and the other, who was the tribal record keeper, had 1.50D. On the other hand, more than 60 percent of the children showed significant amounts of myopia! Obviously they didn't inherit it, and since they were eating the same basic Eskimo food as their parents, it couldn't be explained by nutritional factors. Young concluded that the long periods spent reading schoolwork had caused the myopia.

This conclusion was confirmed by the fact that the incidence of myopia among the Eskimo children was almost identical to that among mainstream American children who were also going through school. Although many scientists had previously cast doubts on the genetic theory, this was the first conclusive proof that heredity is not the major factor. Since Young's discovery, a tremendous amount of supporting evidence has been gained, and it is now known that most common visual problems are not inherited but are caused by environmental factors.

BANKRUPTING THE GENETIC THEORY

Since almost everyone is born with normal healthy eyes, what the genetic theory basically proposes is that millions of normal healthy American children are mysteriously mutating into genetically deformed adults. Fortunately, there's no precedent for such a bizarre phenomenon. Normal healthy children never grow up to develop common genetic deformities such as clubbed feet or cleft palates, and there's no reason to suppose that the eyeballs are an exception to this rule.

Can you imagine the panic that would ensue if millions of normal healthy children started mysteriously mutating into club-footed adults? Do you think that those afflicted would be satisfied if the doctors merely blamed it on genetics and said that nothing could be done except wear special shoes for the rest of their lives, and that they would require larger sizes every few years as the problem got steadily worse? The scenario is so absurd that it hardly bears consideration.

Likewise, the predictions made by the genetic theory fail to pass the test. First, if poor vision is genetic in origin, it shouldn't change after the person becomes an adult because the shape of the eyeballs would be determined by the bone structure of the eyesocket, which is immutable. The truth is that many people with poor vision, especially myopes, often need to change their prescription as adults. If they use traditional eye care they need stronger lenses, whereas if they use vision therapy they need weaker lenses.

Second, it's been found that since the widespread use of computers, millions of adults with normal healthy vision start to develop myopia over the age of thirty, which is long after the point at which the body stops growing. In most of these cases, there is no family history of myopia, so it can't be inherited. Likewise, the genetic structure of a group of people whose only common denominator is that they use a computer can't suddenly change in a single generation, unless computers are mysteriously mutating the eyes. However, if that were true, computer users would also develop longer noses, thicker lips, and bigger ears, which doesn't happen either.

Third, the statistical evidence fails to support the genetic theory. In 1950 a U.S. government study found that the incidence of myopia in the United States was approximately 15 percent of the total population. According to previous reports, this level had remained fairly constant since the 1920s. By 1980, the level had shot up to epidemic proportions of approximately 40 percent. Heredity can't account for the sudden increase because inherited characteristics require many millennia to become dominant in a large population. Young believes that the driving force behind the epidemic was the introduction of television in 1955, which caused millions of people to spend long periods of time focusing close up.

These and other examples have totally demolished the credibility of the genetic theory, and those who are familiar with the evidence regard it as intellectually bankrupt. The question remains, why is a bankrupt theory still taught in medical schools and optometric colleges? The answer lies not in scientific truth but in economics. To put it bluntly, if poor vision is genetic in origin, nothing can be done except prescribe an endless supply of "corrective" lenses, which guarantees eye doctors a lucrative repeat business as patients come back for stronger prescriptions. On the contrary, if poor vision is caused by environmental factors, eye doctors would have a responsibility to try to prevent it, or at least prevent it from becoming worse. This would undermine the foundation of traditional eye care. Hence most eye doctors are either unaware of or refuse to accept the evidence, even though it is abundant, well documented, and persuasive.

FACTORS THAT CAUSE POOR VISION

Since most common visual problems aren't inherited, what are the major causes? We've already discussed developmental visual problems, which usually take the form of poor eye movements, convergence difficulties, lack of depth perception, and lazy or crossed eyes. These problems are very common. In fact, most people have a dominant eye. Several other factors have been identified:

- *The aging process:* This affects the inner lens and all the eye muscles. As a result, accommodation declines and the flow of nutrients is reduced. The most common age-related visual disorders are presbyopia, glaucoma, cataract, and macular degeneration.

- *Iatrogenic problems:* These are secondary problems, especially the loss of natural focusing power, resulting from the use of "corrective" lenses.

• *Stress and posture:* It's well known that stress can affect our bodies in many ways, and the eyes are no exception. The most common stress-related visual problems are eyestrain and myopia. Likewise, bad posture can throw the extraocular muscles out of balance, often causing astigmatism.

Now let's explore the stress factor in more detail.

NEARPOINT STRESS AND MYOPIA

The main characteristic of myopia is that distant objects are blurred although close objects can be seen clearly. If you're a myope, your "corrective" lenses will be minus lenses. To verify this, hold them a few inches above a page of printed material. The letters seen through the lens should be smaller than the letters on the page.

In nature, the price of safety is eternal vigilance. That's why almost all animals and birds constantly look into the distance for signs of danger. Human vision evolved with a similar purpose. Because our ancestors were hunters and warriors, the major biological function of the eyes is to scan the horizon for predators and prey. Hence the anatomy of the eye is specifically structured for long periods of distance vision, together with the ability to focus on close objects for short periods of time. When you read, use a computer, or do any other type of close work for hours at a time, you're using your eyes exactly opposite to the way nature intended. As a result, the visual system becomes stressed and can malfunction. The technical term for this is *nearpoint stress.*

The situation is similar to any other natural bodily action. If you raise your arm for a few seconds, you won't experience any problems. But if you hold it up for several minutes, you'll feel the stress. Your muscles will start to cramp and you'll experience fatigue and eventually some pain. Likewise, the eye muscles respond to long periods of close work by cramping. This is initially experienced as eyestrain, often accompanied by headaches, double vision, and a decrease in tear fluid production, which causes the eyes to become dry, red, and often quite painful.

As the nearpoint stress continues, the eye muscles eventually adapt to the situation. The ciliary muscles lock each eye's inner lens into the bulging accommodated state so that they focus on close objects more easily. Likewise, the extraocular muscles lock the eyeballs into the convergent state so that they point at close objects more easily. Because the eye muscles have changed their configuration to function more efficiently at close range, the ability to focus on distant objects is reduced and the person becomes myopic.

TREATING THE SYMPTOMS AGGRAVATES THE PROBLEM

Statistics reveal that myopes are approximately six times more likely to develop serious eye diseases such as glaucoma, retinal detachment, and cataract. *Hence myopia should not be regarded as a minor social or cosmetic inconvenience but as a potentially blinding disorder.* Unfortunately, because of the limited training they receive at college, the vast majority of traditional eye doctors don't realize the danger and only treat the symptoms by prescribing "corrective" lenses to bring distant objects back into focus.

This method of treatment usually aggravates the problem by creating more nearpoint stress, which causes more myopia and more loss of distance vision. The eye doctor then prescribes even stronger "corrective" lenses, and so on. In this way, patients become trapped in a vicious cycle of progressive myopia and stronger "corrective" lenses, often ending up under the surgeon's knife.

Fortunately, there's a better way. Behavioral optometrists have found that vision therapy and the use of special lenses can usually prevent myopia from occurring in the first place. If myopia is already present, it's often possible to prevent it from progressing and even reverse or eliminate it altogether. We'll discuss these options in more detail later.

POSTURE AND ASTIGMATISM

Astigmatism is a condition in which the eyeball and/or cornea are warped, distorting and blurring the image on the retina. In some cases, the distortion is like looking in a carnival mirror that makes people appear to be abnormally tall and thin or short and fat. Astigmatism usually decreases acuity at all distances and occurs alone or in combination with other visual problems.

If you have astigmatism, your "corrective" lenses will contain what is known as a *cylinder*. To verify this, hold them a few inches above a page of printed material, then rotate them. The letters should become taller and narrower, then shorter and wider. The direction with the letters taller and narrower is called the *axis*. If you have graded bifocals, look for this effect through the top of the lens.

As with myopia, the genetic theory fails to account for the observed facts. If astigmatism is caused by a deformed eyesocket, it would remain constant because the size and shape of the eyesocket doesn't change. The truth is that both the amount of astigmatism and the axis can rapidly change and reverse direction, especially after a neck injury. In fact, chiropractors often report that patients who suffer whiplash in automobile accidents develop astigmatism within a few hours!

Although astigmatism is usually not genetic in origin, it can result from a difficult birth in which the skull and eyesockets become permanently elongated as the baby is squeezed out. This type of person usually has a long narrow face and the astigmatism has a vertical axis. In most cases, however, astigmatism is simply caused by a bad posture with the head habitually tilted to one side.

What is the explanation? One of the visual system's functions is to maintain our sense of balance. Whether we're sitting, standing, or moving, our eyes are constantly scanning the world for signs of the horizontal because we must be aware of the horizontal at all times to avoid falling over. The extraocular muscles are attached to the eyeball in such a way as to facilitate this horizontal scanning movement. When the head is habitually tilted to one side, usually the result of a bad posture, the extraocular muscles adapt by pulling unequally, causing the eyeball and/or cornea to buckle and warp.

Astigmatism is probably the most common visual defect because few people have perfect posture. In most cases, the amount of astigmatism is small and doesn't cause much loss of acuity. On the other hand, heavy readers who habitually tilt their heads often have large amounts of astigmatism combined with myopia. Postural astigmatism is usually not permanent and can often be reduced or eliminated simply by correcting the posture, especially in conjunction with vision therapy.

HYPEROPIA, PRESBYOPIA, AND THE AGING PROCESS

The main characteristic of hyperopia is that close objects are blurred although distant objects can usually be seen clearly. If you're hyperobic, your "corrective" lenses will be plus lenses. To verify this, hold them a few inches above a page of printed material. The letters seen through the lens should be bigger than the letters on the page.

Many people confuse hyperopia with presbyopia. Hyperopia is usually inherited whereas presbyopia is the loss of focusing power associated with the aging process. Most people over forty with otherwise normal vision must hold printed material farther away to see it clearly. As with hyperopia, the traditional remedy for presbyopia is to treat the symptoms with plus lenses, which usually cause dependency and make the eyes lose even more of their natural focusing power, so that stronger prescriptions are needed, thereby trapping patients in a vicious cycle similar to progressive myopia.

People with preexisting visual problems such as astigmatism or myopia also develop presbyopia as they become older. In these cases, the traditional method of treatment is to treat the symptoms with bifocals or trifocals, which also rob the eye of its natural focusing power.

As the inner lens loses its flexibility and the eye muscles lose their strength, focusing becomes sluggish, eye coordination deteriorates, and near objects become blurred. An insidious aspect of presbyopia is that the circulation of blood and nutrients in and around the eyes also declines, increasing the risk of cataracts, macular degeneration, glaucoma, and dry eye syndrome.

USE IT OR LOSE IT

Presbyopia is part of the aging process and affects everyone. There's no escape: you can run but you can't hide. Sooner or later, the aging process catches up with us all and takes its toll. Therein lies an important point: later rather than sooner. There are two types of people. The first type throw up their hands in despair when they turn forty and complain that there's nothing they can do except passively resign themselves to deterioration and senility. They become lazy and neglect their health. Eventually, their negative attitude becomes a self-fulfilling prophecy.

The other type resist the aging process. When they turn forty, they realize that life is a "use it or lose it" situation and that by staying physically active, they can maintain good health and retain their faculties much longer than was previously thought possible. If they're not already leading a healthy lifestyle, they take up some form of moderate exercise such as walking, swimming, or aerobics.

Previous generations were doomed to silently suffer the slings and arrows of outrageous fortune, to patiently endure the whips and scorns of time, anxiously awaiting the grisly grasp of the Grim Reaper. Today, we have the knowledge and power to delay his arrival. One of the most exciting discoveries of this century is that by making a few simple changes, we can grow old gracefully instead of becoming senile and decrepit.

The situation is like tuning up an automobile engine. A new car will run well for about 40,000 miles before showing the first signs of aging. Then the engine won't run as smooth and will burn more fuel. You have a choice. You can say: *"To heck with it, I'll just put on a new muffler and fill up more often."* If that's all the care you give your car, the engine will soon develop serious problems, such as blowing a gasket or burning out the main bearings.

The other choice is to give it a tune-up. By having the engine adjusted, it will run smoothly again and give you many more years of reliable service. The same principle applies to the eyes. We can give the visual system a good tune-up with vision therapy and help it function better. Although we probably won't see as well as we did twenty years ago, we can usually reduce our dependency on "corrective" lenses and delay the need for stronger prescriptions.

CROSSED AND LAZY EYES

These developmental visual problems usually arise during the first few months of life. As we learn to operate the visual system, our brains develop the neural connections that make the eyes work together as a team so that they point at the same object at the same time. If one of the eyes doesn't receive enough visual stimulation during this critical phase, the brain doesn't develop the proper connections and may suppress the image from that eye, making it weak and lazy.

This problem is known as *amblyopia* and can be caused by putting the baby in a crib next to a wall or covering one eye with a blanket for long periods of time. In such an environment, one eye sees a bright new world of moving shapes and colors whereas the other eye just sees the wall or blanket. The result is a highly dominant eye through which the brain does most of its seeing and a lazy eye that the brain ignores. In most cases, there's nothing basically wrong with the lazy eye.

The amblyopic visual system is significantly out of balance, like a four-cylinder engine with two cylinders misfiring. Most of the power is generated by the two good cylinders. Such an automobile won't go very fast and will consume lots of fuel because it's so inefficient. Likewise, people with amblyopia often have other developmental visual problems, such as defective eye movements, poor eye coordination, and reading disabilities.

In minor cases of amblyopia, the brain learns how to coordinate the eyes, but it partially suppresses the lazy eye so that the perceived image is out of focus or fainter than the image from the dominant eye. In major cases where the visual system is severely out of balance, the brain hasn't learned how to coordinate the eyes, which point in different directions. This condition is called *strabismus,* commonly known as crossed eyes.

THE GENETIC THEORY DEBUNKED AGAIN

Many traditional eye doctors, especially ophthalmologists, regard strabismus as a genetic defect. They have been taught that one of the extraocular muscles is attached to the wrong position on the eyeball and causes the eye to point in the wrong direction. Hence they treat strabismus by surgically reattaching the "defective" muscle to a new position. Unfortunately, strabismus surgery is not very effective, with a success rate of only 20 percent. In most cases, the eyes remain straight for a few months, then become crossed again, requiring several more operations. Even worse, strabismus surgery sometimes pinches the vagus nerve, causing cardiac arrest and death.

According to the genetic theory, a single operation should leave the eyes permanently straightened. It is therefore difficult to understand how ophthalmologists can support this theory when they know that several operations are usually needed, unless they seek to profit from the multiple surgeries. Additional evidence that the genetic theory is wrong comes from research where scientists deliberately created strabismus in normal monkeys by surgically reattaching an extraocular muscle to the wrong place. To their amazement, they found that it was impossible to produce a permanent state of strabismus and all the monkeys spontaneously straightened their eyes within a few weeks!

Minor cases of amblyopia and strabismus can often be cured with an eyepatch and vision therapy, and we'll explain how to do this later. More severe cases require the use of lenses containing prisms and other specialized equipment under the care of a behavioral optometrist.

THE TRUTH SHALL SET YOU FREE

In this chapter, we've criticized the genetic theory of poor vision, not because we're opposed to traditional eye doctors, who are usually just repeating what they've been taught at optometric college or medical school, but because there's an abundance of good scientific evidence that convincingly points to environmental factors as the major cause of most common visual problems. This is vitally important because, if visual problems are not genetically determined, they can usually be improved.

But, you may ask, "*What if my parents are myopic and I'm myopic too? Doesn't that mean my myopia is inherited?*" The answer is probably not. In most cases where myopia runs in families, everyone in the family does a lot of reading or close work, which is the common factor causing the myopia, not genetics. As a general rule, inherited visual problems almost always appear early in life. If you had good vision as a child, it's highly unlikely that your visual problem is inherited.

Professor Young explains, "*Just because parents and children speak the same language doesn't mean that language is inherited. The transmission of language results from the fact that parents and children are exposed to the same culture. Likewise, most visual problems, especially myopia, result from the fact that parents and children are exposed to the same environmental influences. Our research clearly shows that excessive close work is the dominant factor in most cases of myopia.*"

HOW TO READ YOUR PRESCRIPTION

By now you should have a good idea of what's really wrong with your eyes. Although vision therapy can improve just about any common visual problem, by understanding your visual problem you'll get the most benefit from the AVI Program and will be able to communicate more effectively with your eye doctor. We also suggest you obtain a copy of your prescription. The following examples will teach you how to read it:

EXAMPLE 1

SACRAMENTO VISIONCARE
OPTOMETRIC CENTER
1111 Howe Ave., Suite 235
Sacramento, California 95825

DAVID W. MURIS, O.D.
Director
Lc. #5059

DALE A. FAST, O.D.
Lc. #4819

GARY K. SCHEFFEL, O.D.
Lc. #5766

Patient ... John Public .... Date ... 3-1-95 ....

℞

OD	−3.50	−.75	x 180	ADD	
OS	−4.00	−1.00	x 5	ADD	PD 64

OD stands for the Latin words *Oculus Dexter* and refers to the right eye. OS stands for *Oculus Sinister* and refers to the left eye. Don't confuse OD with the O.D. found after an optometrist's name, which stands for Doctor of Optometry. If both eyes are the same, OD and OS are often replaced by OU, which stands for *Oculus Uterque*.

The first number following OD or OS refers to the power of the lens in diopters. The larger the number, the stronger the lens. In this example, John Public will receive a −3.50D lens for his right eye and a −4.00D lens for his left eye. The minus signs mean he is myopic and that the left eye is worse than the right.

The next numbers are OD -.75 × 180 and OS −1.00 × 5, which indicate that he has astigmatism in each eye. The −.75 and −1.00 refer to the power of the cylinder, the 180 and 5 refer to the axis. Finally, PD stands for pupillary distance and indicates that the distance between the center of the pupils is 64 mm. This number enables the lenses to be put in the frame so that the center of the lens is aligned with the center of the pupil.

EXAMPLE 2

SACRAMENTO VISIONCARE
OPTOMETRIC CENTER
1111 Howe Ave., Suite 235
Sacramento, California 95825

DAVID W. MURIS, O.D.
Director
Lc. #5059

DALE A. FAST, O.D.
Lc. #4819

GARY K. SCHEFFEL, O.D.
Lc. #5766

Patient ... Jane People .... **Date** ... 3/1/95 ....

℞

OD +1.00   ADD +1.75
                              PD 64/60
OS Plano   ADD +1.75

In this example, Jane People is a presbyope who is being fitted with bifocals. She will receive a +1.00D lens for her right eye and a zero (plano) lens for her left eye. There is no astigmatism. These lenses will form the upper part of the bifocal and indicate that she has lost some distance acuity in her right eye. The numbers following ADD refer to the lower part of the bifocal and mean that both eyes will receive a lens for reading that is +1.75D stronger than the top lens. In other words, the right eye will receive a +2.75D reading lens and the left eye will receive +1.75D reading lens. Jane has a PD of 64/60, which means that the pupillary distance is 64 mm when looking far away and 60 mm with the eyes converged at the normal reading distance of 16 inches.

Of course, some prescriptions are more complicated than these, especially with lenses containing a prism. Contact lens prescriptions also include the curvature of the cornea. However, by studying these examples and comparing them with your own prescription, you should be able to figure out what's wrong with your eyes. If in doubt ask your eye doctor and be on guard if he or she insists that your visual problem is inherited and that nothing can be done about it.

SOME FACTS ABOUT EYE DISEASE

Finally, we'd like to share some sobering statistics about eye disease. According to the National Eye Institute, approximately 15 million Americans over sixty have cataracts, 3 million have glaucoma, and 9 million have some form of retinal degeneration. To put it bluntly, if you rely on traditional eye care, there's almost a 40 percent probability that you'll develop one of these diseases as you grow older. These odds are even worse than Russian roulette, and you should do everything possible to minimize the risk.

This is not a laughing matter. Although many eye doctors don't like to discuss these statistics openly, we believe that patients have the right to know the facts so that they can make informed decisions. In the old days, patients had no choice but to obediently follow "doctor's orders," regardless of the consequences. Today you have a choice and it's important that you clearly understand the alternatives now available to you.

Don't make the mistake of assuming that you'll always be able to see. Really effective eye care is much more than just selecting fashionable frames to go with your next pair of stronger lenses, or assuming that if you develop an eye disease, drugs or surgery will fix it. Although traditional eye care has helped millions of people lead more productive lives, and will continue to play an important role for those who just want a "quick fix," much more can be done. Really effective eye care means spending a few minutes every day exercising your eyes, just like you spend a few minutes every day cleaning your teeth and brushing your hair. It makes a lot of sense and it works.

VISION THERAPY
ALTERNATIVES

TUNING UP THE VISUAL SYSTEM

Suppose you sprained your ankle and your doctor told you that you would be helplessly dependent on crutches for the rest of your life. Even worse, you would probably end up confined to a wheelchair and there was a 40 percent probability that your feet would eventually have to be amputated. Would you accept that diagnosis and obediently follow that method of treatment? Of course you wouldn't! You would insist on doing physical therapy to get your ankle working properly again.

A similar situation exists in traditional eye care but with a major difference. Patients are not told what is really happening to them, neither are they informed about vision therapy. They are merely told that nothing can be done except resign themselves to a lifetime of helpless dependency on progressively stronger "eyecrutches," often followed by surgery as their eyes become ruined. In most cases, no attempt is made to prevent the visual problem or even stop it from getting worse.

The truth is that, like most other parts of the body, the performance of the eyes can be improved by exercise. Dozens of simple techniques have been developed that can help people of all ages enjoy better vision, healthier eyes, and a happier and more productive lifestyle. Eye exercises, commonly known as *vision therapy*, encompass a wide range of techniques that make the visual system more efficient. Some techniques improve eye coordination and increase the power of the focusing system. Other techniques reduce visual stress and promote the flow of nutrients to the eyes, making them healthier and more relaxed.

The AVI Program will give your eyes a good basic workout. In contrast to physical exercises, eye exercises are not strenuous and are concerned with increasing the power and accuracy of the focusing system rather than beefing up the eye muscles. Although your eyes will become "stronger," the process is like making an engine more powerful by tuning it up and using better fuel. Technical details are given in the Appendix.

If you do the AVI Program exactly as directed and don't take shortcuts, you should see significant results within a month. Typical areas of improvement are listed below and will give you a realistic idea of what can be achieved. Of course, not everyone will improve in all these areas and the actual results will vary from person to person depending on the severity of the condition, state of health, lifestyle, stress level, diet, and degree of compliance.

- Stronger eyes with more natural focusing power

- Healthier eyes with less risk of major eye diseases

- Reduce or eliminate dependency on "corrective" lenses

- Prevent further deterioration and avoid stronger prescriptions

- More comfortable, relaxed vision with better eye coordination

- Relief from computer-induced headaches and eyestrain

- Improve dry eyes and reduce sensitivity to bright light

- Faster reading and better comprehension

Although many people see the first signs of improvement within a week, don't be impatient or discouraged if you don't get astonishing results right away. Remember that we're doctors, not miracle workers. So be realistic. If you've worn "corrective" lenses for many years, don't expect your vision to clear up overnight. Give the therapy time to work and don't expect too much too soon. Although some people do get exciting results very quickly, the rate of improvement is usually more gradual. The important thing is to patiently persevere and remember that positive actions *must* produce positive results.

CLUSTERS OF HABIT PATTERNS

Fortunately, we've developed some simple techniques that will enable you to exercise your eyes every day without taking up any extra time, even if you have a busy schedule. It is truly said that man is a creature of habit. In fact, the majority of our actions are governed by clusters of habit patterns that help us do ordinary things without constantly having to make decisions. Instead of consciously calculating every single action, we rely on habit patterns to help us live automatically without really thinking about what we're doing.

Almost everything we do on a regular basis is habitual. For example, driving a car is a cluster of habit patterns. We automatically step on the gas pedal, look in the mirror, use the turn signals, move the steering wheel, and apply the brakes as needed. We don't have to think about these actions. We just do them subconsciously. How many times have you passed a highway exit because your mind was a million miles away and you were just driving habitually?

Likewise, we rely on clusters of habit patterns to operate our visual systems. Imagine how complicated life would be if we had to consciously calculate the position of every object we wanted to look at, make the appropriate eye movements, calculate the distance of the object, then focus the eyes! Not suprisingly, the majority of people with poor eyesight have bad visual habits. Most nearsighted people habitually read or work at a computer hour after hour without stopping or looking away, so that their eyes become strained. Likewise, most people who wear "corrective" lenses habitually leave them on all the time, so that they become dependent on them.

If you seriously want to improve your eyesight, you must carefully cultivate the New Visual Habits outlined in Chapter 4 until they are completely automatic. Truly effective habits are firmly embedded in the subconscious, therefore you must resolutely repeat your New Visual Habits over and over again until they become part of your normal way of seeing.

MAKE A FORMAL DECISION TO SUCCEED

The first and most important step in developing your New Visual Habits is to sincerely believe that you need to make some positive changes. This means weighing the pros and cons and making an intelligent choice so that you're convinced you're doing the right thing. Just as the road to hell is paved with good intentions, it's probably true that in many cases the road to blindness is paved with "corrective" lenses. We'll discuss the harmful effects of "corrective" lenses in more detail later. For now, recognize the fact that traditional eye care is leading you on a downward spiral into stronger prescriptions and you must turn things around before its too late.

The next step is to make a formal decision that nothing will stop you from succeeding. Make a solemn vow or written contract with yourself that you're going to succeed. Then make your decision public by telling your friends and coworkers. A public commitment is important because it makes you accountable to other people. If you make a secret contract with yourself, you can always find some excuse to wriggle out of it. Although you may experience a few pangs of guilt and remorse, your "solid decision" will be quickly forgotten and you'll just continue to deteriorate as your old visual habits reassert themselves.

So don't let yourself fail. Make a public commitment and put the AVI Program into action. Remember, all new habits take about a month to become firmly established. During this period you may experience some resistance from your old visual habits, which just want to be left alone. Don't let bad thoughts or feelings stop you from succeeding! Do whatever it takes to firmly establish your New Visual Habits!

OPPORTUNITIES FOR ACTION

Now let's get into specifics. Your New Visual Habits consist of some simple therapy techniques to integrate with your normal activities until exercising your eyes becomes totally automatic and you don't have to think about it. Practice these techniques on the world around you until they become part of your normal way of seeing. Starting today, practice your New Visual Habits as often as possible when working, waiting, driving, using the phone, reading, using a computer, or during TV commercials. You'll find plenty of opportunities. The techniques involve only eye movements so they're invisible to others. You can do them in a room full of people and nobody will realize what you're doing!

Please don't complain that you don't have enough time. *The good news is that your New Visual Habits won't take up any extra time because you'll be doing these things anyway.* You'll simply use your time more productively. In fact, your New Visual Habits will make boring activities more interesting because you'll develop a better way of seeing. And remember, the payoff is a lifetime of brighter, clearer vision.

THE YEAR OF TRAFFIC LIGHTS

The time spent waiting at traffic lights provides most people with the best opportunity for everyday practice. The average person stops at about ten traffic lights per day and wastes a minute or two at each light. This can add up to twenty minutes a day, or more than a year during your entire lifetime. Imagine spending a whole year waiting for the lights to change! You're stuck in your car and there's no escape. You can't avoid them and they're only going to become more numerous as the city expands. So what are you going to do? Are you going to desperately pound your fists on the steering wheel and drive yourself into a frenzied fit of anger and frustration?

Not anymore! From this day forth and for the rest of your life, practice your New Visual Habits every time you stop at a traffic light until they become an integral part of your normal driving routine. Just as you automatically use the brake pedal to stop, you should automatically do some vision therapy every time you wait for a light to change. Use your valuable time productively instead of wasting it.

THE THREE PHASES OF VISION THERAPY

The most important thing is to generate momentum and enthusiasm as quickly as possible. Get up to speed and *see* the results! That's the key to success. Once you actually *see* the difference for yourself, you'll know beyond a shadow of doubt that you've made the right decision. You'll experience such a tremendous feeling of satisfaction and accomplishment that you'll never look back! You'll never want to go back to dependency on "corrective" lenses, trapped in the vicious cycle of weaker eyes and stronger prescriptions!

Vision therapy can be a lot of fun as you see the techniques work for you day after day. You'll soon develop a bright new view of the world that will forever change the way you use your eyes. Although many people see the first signs of improvement in a few days, the major goal of the therapy is to produce positive long-term changes. You'll probably find that your vision will pass through several phases as it improves:

PHASE 1: LEARNING

During the first couple of weeks, your goal is to become thoroughly familiar with all the techniques so that you can do them without referring to the book. We suggest you read the instructions for each technique three times to make sure you don't miss anything. Follow the method exactly as directed. In addition to the New Visual Habits, we've provided you with some Booster Sequences that you should do for ½ hour a day for a month.

Reduce your dependency on "corrective" lenses as quickly as possible unless your goal is to stabilize your vision, in which case just concentrate on seeing more clearly through your current prescription.

PHASE 2: DEVELOPMENT

This is a period of rapid progress that usually lasts from one to three months, depending on the visual problem. Your goal is to build momentum and get as much improvement as possible. You'll master all the techniques and will figure out which are working best for you. You'll go from one weaker prescription to the next and reduce your dependency on "corrective" lenses even further. You'll be practicing your New Visual Habits on a regular basis and they'll become part of your normal way of seeing.

Most people report that it takes only a few weeks to adapt to a weaker prescription, sometimes only a few days. Once you've adapted to a weaker prescription, move on to the next weaker prescription as quickly as possible. During this phase, you may also experience *clear flashes,* which are periods of clear vision without "corrective" lenses. These are quite common and have even been reported by people with really poor vision. With perseverance, the clear flashes usually become longer and more intense. However, not everyone gets them, so don't be disappointed if you don't. The usual rate of progress is more gradual, improving from one weaker prescription to the next.

PHASE 3: MAINTENANCE

Most people eventually reach a plateau where no more improvement takes place or the rate of improvement is so slow they decide to stop doing the Booster Sequences. When you reach this plateau, your New Visual Habits will be so firmly established that they should automatically maintain the results and continue the improvement at a more gradual rate. *However, this plateau probably doesn't represent the maximum amount of improvement possible!*

Many people find that this plateau is only temporary and that if they continue to do the Booster Sequences on a regular basis as part of their health and fitness routine, their vision eventually goes through another burst of improvement and reaches another plateau. Then the same thing happens: another period of consolidation followed by another burst of improvement.

The consolidation-improvement cycle can continue for a long time and offers hope that even people with serious visual problems can eventually return to normal. The key is to develop the habit of doing some vision therapy every day so that it becomes an integral part of your lifestyle. Whether it takes a month or a year to return to normal, it doesn't really matter because you've made a long-term commitment to give your eyes the special care and attention they deserve. Just keep doing the therapy on a regular basis and have confidence in your body's ability to heal itself.

POSITIVE CHANGES MUST TAKE PLACE

As the therapy takes effect, positive changes will occur in the shape and structure of your eyes. These changes are inevitable because the eyes are part of the body and they obey the same laws of physics and muscular development. It's an established fact that if you exercise your body on a regular basis, positive changes will take place in its shape and structure. Likewise, because vision therapy improves the power and coordination of the eye muscles and increases the nutrient flow, these forces *must* produce positive changes at a cellular level and ultimately at a structural level. The laws of nature must be obeyed!

The plateaus and consolidation periods appear to represent the time needed for these structural changes to take place. So don't get discouraged and think you've reached your limit and nothing more will happen. Many positive changes are happening as the cells regroup and regenerate the tissues. Even with cataracts or macular degeneration, a lot can be done to improve the flow of nutrients. Many people with serious problems have achieved major improvements, and there's no reason why you shouldn't, too. Don't limit yourself with negative self-fulfilling prophecies. Don't expect miracles, but don't set yourself up for failure.

Fortunately, the eyes are not rigidly backed up against a wall of bone. The eyeball is separated from the eyesocket by about ½ inch of fatty tissue, which allows plenty of room for changes to take place. That's why even people with serious problems can achieve major results. Approximately 2 million cells die every second and are replaced by new cells. The structure of the body constantly changes. Nothing remains the same, even for a moment. The AVI Program will direct these changes toward better vision. Just develop the habit of doing some therapy on a regular basis and your vision will improve of its own accord.

4

SEVEN NEW VISUAL HABITS

BUILD A SOLID FOUNDATION

The following seven simple New Visual Habits form the foundation of our method. Pumping and Tromboning exercise the focusing mechanism and stimulate the flow of nutrients inside the eyes. Clock Rotations and Eye Rolls stimulate the flow of nutrients around the eyeball and improve control of the extraocular muscles. Slow Blinking reduces visual stress. Squeeze Blinking stimulates the production of tear fluid. Blur Zoning sharpens acuity by improving the ability to see small details.

These techniques will give your eyes and surrounding tissues a good basic workout. The beauty of the method is that it doesn't take any extra time. It gradually improves almost any common visual problem, regardless of age or circumstances. It allows you to give your eyes some real care and attention instead of just letting them get worse.

As a bonus, you should become a safer driver because you'll pay more attention to other vehicles and the world around you. There are some other important techniques that we'll discuss later that you should do on a daily basis for about a month, but the bottom line is to image starts to break up or go out of focus. Don't do this technique quickly. The most important thing is to keep the image single and in focus as long as possible. You should also move the object very slowly as you take it away from your nose. Myopes may find that the object will go out of focus very close to their nose and also before they reach arm's length. The same principle applies. Keep it single and in focus as long as possible, whatever the distance.

NEW VISUAL HABIT #3: CLOCK ROTATIONS

Look at a far object directly ahead and imagine that you're in front of a giant clock with the far object at the center. Keep your head and shoulders still and carefully move your eyes as far as they will go in the 9 o'clock direction as though you're trying to see your left ear. Keep the extraocular muscles fully stretched for a couple of seconds and don't look at anything in particular. Then return to the far object at the center.

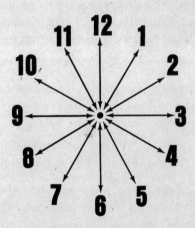

Now carefully move the eyes as far as they will go in the 10 o'clock direction for a couple of seconds as though you're trying to see just above your left ear and gently stretch the extraocular muscles. Then return to the far object at the center. Now the 11 o'clock direction, then the far object at the center. Don't do this technique quickly. Continue to slowly make your way around the clock, carefully moving the eyes as far as they will go in the direction of each number, stretching the extraocular muscles, then returning to the far object at the center:

(9/stretch) (center) (10/stretch) (center) (11/stretch) (center) (12/stretch) (center) and so on.

NEW VISUAL HABIT #4: EYE ROLLS

Slowly roll your eyes in a complete circle, first one way then the other, keeping the extraocular muscles fully stretched at all times. Don't do this technique quickly. The important thing is coordination and control, so aim for slow, smooth rotations without jerkiness or looking at anything in particular.

Some words of caution regarding Clock Rotations and Eye Rolls. Although you should stretch the extraocular muscles as far as they will go, don't violently jerk them or stretch them so hard that you see flashes of light. If this happens, you are stressing the retina. This is especially important for myopes. The goal is to develop smooth, controlled eye movements, not build bigger muscles. So aim for power and control, but don't overdo it.

If you suffer from motion sickness you may find that Clock Rotations and Eye Rolls make you dizzy. If this happens, cover your eyes with your hands and do them with your eyes open underneath.

NEW VISUAL HABIT #5: SLOW BLINKING

Breathe slowly and deeply. As you inhale, don't look at anything in particular but just do a few normal blinks and fill your lungs completely. As you exhale, close your eyes, relax, and slowly blow all the air out of your lungs while mentally or verbally repeating: "Relax! Relax! Relax!" While exhaling, don't do anything with your eyes. No eye movements or squeezing. Just keep them gently closed and relaxed. Continue to Slow Blink in time to your breathing:

(inhale/open) (exhale/relax) (inhale/open) (exhale/relax) (inhale/open) (exhale/relax) and so on.

New Visual Habit #6: Squeeze Blinking

Squeeze your eyelids tightly shut and hold to a count of three. Then open your eyes wide and do a few normal blinks. Then squeeze tightly shut again, then open again. Continue to alternate squeezing and opening. After a few Squeeze Blinks, your eyes will feel pleasantly moist from the production of tear fluid. Isolate the eyelid muscles and don't frown or scrunch up the forehead muscles or the muscles around the eyes: squeeze-open-squeeze-open-squeeze-open-squeeze-open-squeeze-open-squeeze, and so on.

New Visual Habit #7: Blur Zoning

Slowly run your gaze around the edge of a blurred object and follow the major outlines. Don't just stare at the outlines, but move the eyes and follow the edges. For example, if you're myopic, look at a tree and follow the outlines formed by the branches against the sky as you explore the nooks and crannies. If you're hyperopic or presbyopic, distant objects will probably be clear so hold a trinket or piece of jewelry close enough so that it's blurred.

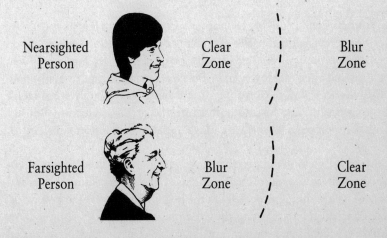

| Nearsighted Person | Clear Zone | | Blur Zone |
| Farsighted Person | Blur Zone | | Clear Zone |

After doing this for a few seconds, carefully study the *smallest detail* you can see and try to determine its exact shape. Then try to see smaller and smaller details, down to the limits of your perception. For example, myopes should look at a cluster of leaves and try to see an individual leaf. Hyperopes and presbyopes should look at fine details on the surface, such as scratch marks or the grain of the metal. Don't squint or use any tricks. Just aim for calm, relaxed, contemplative vision, and carefully pick out smaller and smaller details.

MAKE HASTE SLOWLY AND DON'T OVERDO IT

Don't try to do all the techniques at every traffic light. Rotate them. At one traffic light, do some Pumping. At the next, some Tromboning. At the next, some Slow Blinking. After doing them for a while, you'll find that some of the techniques are more effective than others. Master them all. Then concentrate on the techniques that are giving you the most benefit. If you don't do much driving, practice them during TV commercials or when reading or using the phone. Instead of wasting valuable time channel-hopping or vacantly gazing into space, practice your New Visual Habits. If you do calisthenics, weight training, or walking, you can exercise your eyes at the same time with Pumping, Eye Rolls, or Squeeze Blinking.

Your eyes will probably feel rather sore for the first few days because you're exercising the muscles and giving them a healthy workout. Soon the discomfort will be replaced by positive new feelings of power, vitality, and control. However, if you experience any type of major pain or discomfort, you're overdoing it and must immediately stop! Don't try to force things. Instead, substitute the Stress Reduction Booster Sequences on page 83 for a few days until the discomfort subsides.

Most people don't experience any problems. However, exercise enthusiasts such as weight lifters, gymnasts, or runners should be careful not to overdo things, especially in the beginning. During the first week, just concentrate on learning the eye movements and developing coordination, then build power and stamina. Developing New Visual Habits is like planting seeds. Once they take root, they'll give you a lifetime of healthier eyes and better vision.

HOW TO OVERCOME CONVERGENCE PROBLEMS

Slow readers or people who suffer from motion sickness often have convergence problems and may get headaches from Pumping or Tromboning. If this happens, don't wait for the headache to build up. Immediately stop and do a Slow Blink. Close your eyes and breathe slowly and deeply until the headache goes away. Then do some more Pumping or Tromboning.

When the headache returns, immediately stop and do another Slow Blink. Then continue to Pump or Trombone and try to extend the time by a few seconds. Continue to steadily increase the amount of time and do a Slow Blink whenever the headache returns. In this way, you will gradually work your way through the problem until you can do Pumping or Tromboning without any discomfort whatsoever. This is often accompanied by a major increase in reading speed. In other cases, motion sickness is completely cured.

WEAN YOURSELF FROM "CORRECTIVE" LENSES

As you probably know from your own experience, "corrective" lenses usually cause dependency and make the eyes weaker, so that they lose even more of their natural focusing power. After wearing a new prescription for just a few weeks, most people can't see as well without it as they could before they started wearing it. The problems caused by these products are so widespread that many eye doctors now believe that they can damage the eyes. This warning applies to glasses and contact lenses.

As a general rule, wear them as little as possible and don't just leave them on all the time. Regard them as tools to be used for activities where you *must* have clear vision, and cultivate the habit of removing them as soon as you've finished the activity. Wean yourself from your "eyecrutches" and learn to see for yourself. Remember, if you get headaches without them, you're straining your eyes instead of relaxing and accepting what you can see.

At first, it may be emotionally difficult to go without your "eye-crutches," especially if you've worn them for many years, and some people may panic when they leave them off for the first time. If this happens, do some Slow Blinking and the panic will quickly subside. If you cultivate the habit of leaving them off for longer and longer periods of time, you'll find that there are many situations where you can see well without them, even if things are not perfectly clear. Of course, don't leave them off in potentially dangerous situations, such as driving, cooking, or using power tools.

HOW TO MAXIMIZE HABIT FORMATION

We've summarized your New Visual Habits on the Reminder Page. Remove the page and cut it into two panels. Tape the panel marked "CAR" to your dashboard and use the panel marked "BOOKMARK" for your major reading. Put the Bookmark one page ahead and when you reach it, stop reading and practice your New Visual Habits for a few seconds. This is a great technique for wading through a pile of paperwork.

If you use the phone a lot, tape a Bookmark to it and do vision therapy between calls. For example, a Slow Blink after every call will refresh you and help you work more productively. This is a good way of managing your time so you don't get stressed or burned out. Try it. You'll like it.

Do whatever it takes to remind yourself to do the therapy and firmly establish your New Visual Habits so that you don't have to think about them. Concentrate on getting results as quickly as possible so that you build momentum and enthusiasm. Carefully integrate the techniques with your everyday activities so that you develop "conditioned re-flexes." Then the activities themselves will automatically trigger your New Visual Habits every time they occur.

THE THREE PHASES OF HABIT FORMATION

During the first week, pay special attention to the way your eyes feel and repeatedly remind yourself to do the therapy. Soon, you'll notice the first signs of habit formation. Perhaps you'll be wasting time at a traffic light or channel-hopping and your mind will be a million miles away dreaming about something else.

Suddenly, without even thinking about it, you'll spontaneously do some Pumping or perhaps a Slow Blink. You'll experience a burst of excitement as you realize that your New Visual Habits are starting to take root in your subconscious. As the days go by, you'll find yourself spontaneously practicing your New Visual Habits more and more often.

After about a month, you'll enter another phase. By then your New Visual Habits will be totally automatic and firmly embedded in your subconscious. You'll be doing vision therapy at almost every traffic light, and you'll now make a commitment to keep doing it for the rest of your life.

As you make this commitment, you'll experience a profound sense of accomplishment. Instead of wasting valuable time, you're using it more productively. Instead of helplessly resigning yourself to stronger prescriptions and a 40 percent risk of developing a serious eye disease, you've taken control and changed the course of your life for the better!

LIMITS OF APPLICATION

We must emphasize that the AVI Program is not a "miracle method." If you wear thick glasses, you probably won't be able to throw them away after only a month of therapy. Nevertheless, some people do indeed get "miraculous" results and we don't want to limit you by telling you that it's impossible. The human mind possesses an amazing amount of natural healing power and the AVI Program will teach you how to harness it.

So on one hand we don't want to tell you that you can't throw away your glasses and return to normal. On the other hand, we don't want to fill you up with empty promises and unrealistic expectations so that you become disappointed if it doesn't happen. Take the attitude that you'll expect the best but will settle for less. The truth is that the results vary and some people respond better than others. The only way to find out is to give it your best effort and see for yourself.

GENERAL AREAS OF IMPROVEMENT

Regardless of your age or the severity of your visual problem or the number of years you've worn "corrective" lenses, there are some basic results that most people obtain. Even if you don't reach the stage where you can throw away your "corrective" lenses, you can realistically expect to see more clearly, comfortably, and efficiently.

Because the therapy gives your eye muscles a good basic workout, your eyes will feel more powerful and you'll be able to change focus faster and easier. You'll feel that your eyes are working better, are more responsive, and don't get as tired. Your acuity will improve and you'll be able to see smaller details than before.

Likewise, because the therapy boosts the flow of nutrients to the entire eye region, your eyes will become healthier and will feel more alive. Many people start the therapy with tired, aching eyes and after a month are surprised to find that their eyes actually sparkle with new health and vitality. Dry eye syndrome and sensitivity to bright light often clear up and crow's feet may actually disappear as the nutrient flow rejuvenates the cells and stimulates the skin. The revitalization process can be quite remarkable and is one of the more gratifying aspects of the therapy.

Furthermore, because the therapy brings the visual system into greater balance, many people find that the world appears to be more solid and three-dimensional. Colors may become brighter and more vivid. Reading speed may increase and comprehension may improve. This can translate into better performance at work, school, and sports, and may even lead to a a a higher-paying job.

Finally, because the AVI Program teaches you to use stress-reduction techniques during your normal daily activities, you'll become a more confident and relaxed person who can handle the tensions and anxieties of life more easily. You'll experience a profound feeling of pride and accomplishment because you've done something really good for your eyes instead of just letting them get worse. And you'll have the reassurance of knowing that you've taken major steps to reduce the risk of cataracts and other serious eye diseases.

SET YOURSELF REALISTIC GOALS

The AVI Program is designed to improve eyestrain, astigmatism, myopia, hyperopia, presbyopia, lazy eye, cataracts, and macular degeneration. The following guidelines come from using these techniques in clinical practice with thousands of patients and will give you a realistic idea of what to aim for.

- *If your vision has just started to deteriorate,* you can probably return to normal and avoid "corrective" lenses. If you're over forty and starting to become presbyopic, you may eventually have to wear them as the aging process takes its toll, but you can probably delay them for several years. Minor visual problems such as loss of focusing power, eyestrain, or headaches from using computers usually clear up within a few weeks, sometimes within a few days.

- *If your prescription is weak,* you can probably return to normal or near-normal vision. If you've just started wearing "corrective" lenses, spend as much time as possible without them. If you've progressed to a stronger prescription, go back to wearing your weaker prescription if you still have it. If not, ask your eye doctor for a weaker prescription. You should also reduce your dependency on "corrective" lenses as much as possible.

• *If your prescription is medium or strong,* you can probably gain a substantial amount of freedom from "corrective" lenses. With patience and perseverance, you may eventually get rid of them completely. The key is to adapt to a series of weaker prescriptions. Use weaker glasses or contact lenses from previous years or ask your eye doctor for weaker prescriptions. This strategy is known as *progressive undercorrection* and is the exact opposite of traditional eye care because it uses "corrective" lenses to help patients get better, not worse.

Even with a strong prescription, it's often possible to achieve significant results within a few weeks, although much more therapy is usually needed to obtain the maximum improvement. Concentrate on your New Visual Habits so that time isn't a problem. Remember, even if it takes several months to improve from one weaker prescription to the next, you'll be stopping at hundreds of traffic lights on the way, so make the most of them and use your time productively.

Also reduce your dependency on "corrective" lenses by spending a few hours a day without them instead of habitually leaving them on all the time. Myopes should do as much of their close work as possible without "corrective" lenses and try to use them only for distance vision. Presbyopes should try to avoid bifocals and use only single-vision glasses. The important thing is to make the eyes work and regain as much of your natural focusing power as possible.

• *You can stabilize your vision at its present level,* and avoid the anxiety and expense of a stronger prescription. This usually takes just a few weeks and may be the best course of action for people with really poor vision or those who don't want to do much therapy. Although stabilization doesn't sound very exciting, it's a tremendous accomplishment if your vision has been getting steadily worse for a long time. Many people with thick glasses are justifiably concerned about going blind and are happy just to stop the downhill progression.

• *If you have cataracts or macular degeneration,* you can probably halt or slow down the deterioration. Cataracts are easiest to improve and sometimes clear up completely. Macular degeneration is more difficult to treat and no cure is known, although significant improvements often take place.

LEARN TO SEE FOR YOURSELF

One of the most harmful myths perpetrated by the eye care establishment is that going without "corrective" lenses will damage your eyes. There is not a shred of evidence to support this point of view. On the contrary, spending time without "corrective" lenses is one of the simplest and most effective vision therapy techniques, because it breaks the vicious cycle of dependency and deterioration. Use "corrective" lenses as tools for activities that require clear vision and remove them as soon as you've finished the activity. In summary, we recommend the following strategies:

1. If your prescription is weak and your goal is to return to normal vision, try to do it in one step without getting another weaker prescription. Spend as much time as possible without "corrective" lenses. If you do a lot of reading or computer work, you may find it helpful to use stress-relieving glasses. We'll discuss these later.

2. If your goal is to adapt to a weaker prescription, start wearing it immediately. If you continue to wear your current prescription it will interfere with the therapy and hold you back. A weaker prescription is important because it stimulates the focusing mechanism and exercises your eyes so that they become stronger. The weaker prescription should give you 20/40 acuity in each eye so that objects are rather blurred. When you can see clearly through

the weaker prescription, get another weaker prescription. Continue to adapt to weaker prescriptions until you no longer need them or achieve the maximum amount of improvement possible.

3. If your goal is to stabilize your vision and avoid a stronger prescription, continue to wear your current prescription as usual and simply concentrate on seeing more clearly through it.

SIXTEEN BOOSTER TECHNIQUES

DEVOTE A MONTH TO VISION THERAPY

Although the New Visual Habits form the foundation of our method, there are sixteen other vision therapy techniques that you should learn. These are known as the *Booster Techniques* and should be practiced for ½ hour a day for a month. They are arranged in special sequences known as the *Booster Sequences*.

Please don't resort to the feeble excuse that you don't have enough time. Your eyes must last your entire lifetime, so you owe it to yourself to learn how to take care of them properly. The knowledge you'll gain will yield immediate benefits and will significantly reduce the risk of degenerative eye diseases later in life. You can cut back on TV for a month, can't you? Of course you can! Once you've learned the techniques you can decide if you want to continue. *So do yourself a favor and devote the next thirty days to mastering our method. You'll be glad you did!*

CONTROL YOUR INNER DIALOGUE

Whether you realize it or not, you're mentally talking to yourself most of the time. This inner dialogue is an endless commentary about your life, relationships, feelings, fantasies, problems, and so on. This stream of thoughts and mental images influences your attitudes, actions and entire state of being.

Most people fail to achieve their goals because their inner dialogue is dominated by unproductive thoughts and negative mental images. They just reflect the world around them and are swept along by events and the things they see on TV. Even worse, many people focus on negativity, constantly trying to find excuses, laying blame on others, and avoiding responsibility for their actions. As a result, their negative attitude reinforces the negative events that occur and they become victims of their own creation.

In contrast, most successful people share a common secret. Instead of constantly criticizing and complaining, they control their inner dialogue and use it to consciously direct the course of their life. They don't waste valuable time and energy dwelling on negativity but deliberately generate a steady stream of positive thoughts and actions. They take control of their thoughts, words, and deeds and focus them on their goals.

The biggest obstacle to success is procrastination. If you seriously want to improve your vision, *start doing the therapy today, right now, immediately.* If you procrastinate, you'll have taken your first step on the downward spiral of delays, excuses, forgetfulness, and stronger prescriptions. Make no mistake: the longer you delay, the more likely you are to get sidetracked and forget. The more excuses you make, the easier it is to make them. Even worse, once you forget, you won't even realize you've forgotten. So start practicing the techniques *right now* and focus your mind on getting rapid results!

Now for the Booster Techniques. These will really accelerate your progress, so study them carefully and don't skip anything or take shortcuts. In the next chapter, we'll give you the complete Booster Sequences together with advice for different visual problems. But before proceeding, cut out all the charts at the back of the book with a razor blade or exacto knife. It's a good idea to make photocopies to put on your TV or computer, or on the wall at your workplace.

TECHNIQUE #1: POWER THINKING

For thousands of years it has been known that the mind exerts a powerful effect over the body, and even the medical profession is now recognizing the healing potential of prayer and positive thinking. Your mind is a lot more powerful than you probably realize and you should assertively harness that power to improve your vision.

The best way of doing this is to focus your mental energy with an affirmation. This is a positive statement that embodies your goals. Resolutely repeating an affirmation stimulates natural healing power and builds motivation so that you persevere and get rapid results. Choose one of the affirmations below or invent your own. It doesn't really matter which affirmation you choose as long as you feel comfortable with it. If you are religious, combine it with a prayer. Cultivate the habit of repeating it over and over again until it becomes part of you:

I see better every day!
My vision is improving!
I can see without glasses!
My eyes are getting better!
I have natural healthy vision!
I see distant objects more clearly!
Positive changes are now taking place!
I see clearly, comfortably, and naturally!
My eyes are feeling comfortable and relaxed!
The shape and structure of my eyes is improving!

Verbally repeat it as much as possible during your normal activities, while working, playing, shopping, driving, and so on. Say it aloud when you're alone. Whisper it under your breath when you're with other people. Write it on brightly colored pieces of paper and put them in prominent positions at home, in your car, and at work.

When circumstances permit, repeat it with as much energy as you can muster, even shouting it at the top of your voice. You can also sing or chant it while clapping your hands. The more energy you give it, the more effective it becomes. Get the adrenaline flowing and energize your mind!

TECHNIQUE #2: FAST BLINKING

Breathe slowly and deeply. As you inhale, don't look at anything in particular, just do a few normal blinks and fill your lungs completely. As you exhale, open and close your eyes as quickly as possible and slowly blow all the air out of your lungs. Continue to Fast Blink in time to your breathing:

(inhale/open) (exhale/fast blink) (inhale/open) (exhale/fast blink) (inhale/open) (exhale/fast blink) (inhale/open) and so on.

TECHNIQUE #3: NOSE FUSION

Breathe slowly and deeply. As you inhale, cross your eyes by looking at the tip of your nose. You should be able to see both sides of your nose at the same time. As you exhale, uncross your eyes, look at a distant object, and slowly blow all the air out of your lungs. Continue to slowly cross and uncross your eyes in time to your breathing:

(inhale/cross) (exhale/uncross) (inhale/cross) (exhale/uncross) (inhale/cross) (exhale/uncross) (inhale/cross) and so on.

If you can't do this technique, do Tromboning instead.

TECHNIQUE #4: FUSION CHART

Hold the Fusion Chart at arm's length and look at the top row of faces. Now cross your eyes by looking at the tip of your nose. Then slowly uncross them. The faces should fuse together to form a central face with a fainter face on either side. Another way of doing this is to hold a pencil halfway between the chart and your eyes. When you look at the pencil, the faces should fuse together in the background.

Stabilize the central face by slowly running your gaze around the edges and focusing on details. Now fuse the lower rows of faces.

When you can do this easily, vary the procedure by slowly moving the chart toward you with the faces fused until the central face breaks up.

TECHNIQUE #5: FUSION PUMPING

Once you've mastered the Fusion Chart, you can use it as the near object for Pumping. Fuse the faces and when the central face is stable, look at a far object. Then fuse the central face again. Continue to change focus back and forth between the fused central face and a far object.

TECHNIQUE #6: BLUR READING

Put some reading material upside down, deep into your blur zone. Myopes should use a newspaper or magazine as far away as possible. Presbyopes should use a book less than 3 inches away from the eyes. Now look at any word and slowly run your gaze around it. If you can see the individual letters, slowly run your gaze around them and concentrate on the exact outline of each letter. Then slowly run your gaze around other words.

TECHNIQUE #7: SCANNING CHART

Put the Scanning Chart just into your blur zone so that it's slightly blurred. Now jump from dot to dot and follow the line all the way from A to B, then back again. First the large chart, then the small chart. Spend a couple of seconds on each dot. Every time you do this technique, vary the chart's position so that you don't memorize the pattern. Turn it upside down or put it at an angle. Vary the procedure by putting it deep into your blur zone as with Blur Reading.

TECHNIQUE #8: ACUITY CHART

Put the Acuity Chart just into your blur zone so that it's slightly blurred. Now look at the smallest line you can read and calmly run your gaze back and forth a few times along the line above, which will consist of even smaller words. Then carefully study the outline of one of the words on that line. Breathe slowly, blink frequently, and don't hurry, squint, or stare. When you can read some words on that line, go to the line above and repeat the procedure. Continue to make your way up the chart from one line to the smaller line above. If the entire chart clears up, move it deeper into your blur zone.

TECHNIQUE #9: ACUPRESSURE A

Close your eyes and put your thumbs as shown in the diagram. For most people the acupressure point is a small bony knob or ridge just inside the rim of the eye socket below the eyebrow. The goal is to massage the acupressure point so that it becomes slightly sore without actually hurting. When you find it, you will experience a tender "nervy" feeling. Press firmly for a second, then release for a second. Continue to alternate pressing and releasing without touching the eyeball: press-release-press-release-press-release-press-release-press-release-press-release, and so on.

TECHNIQUE #10: ACUPRESSURE B

Close your eyes and put your thumbs in the pit of your temples. Now firmly stroke the upper rims of your eye sockets using the flat part of your fingers between the first and second joints. Firmly stroke the lower rims of the eye sockets. Continue to alternate stroking the upper, then the lower rims, always going from your nose to the temples. You may find it helpful to use vaseline or vitamin E as a lubricant to avoid stretching the skin: upper-lower-upper-lower-upper-lower-upper-lower-upper-lower-upper-lower, and so on.

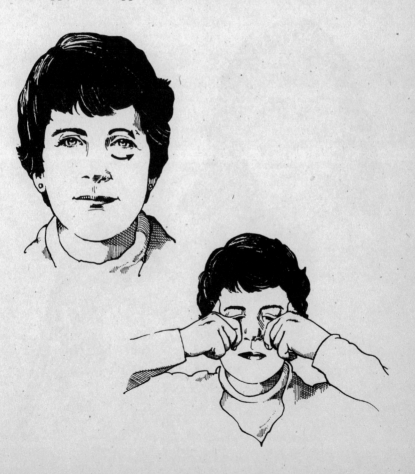

TECHNIQUE #11: ACUPRESSURE C

Close your eyes and position your thumb and index finger as shown in the diagram. Now firmly massage the bridge of your nose by alternate squeezing, then releasing, making it slightly sore without actually hurting: squeeze-release-squeeze-release-squeeze-release-squeeze-release-squeeze, and so on.

TECHNIQUE #12: ACUPRESSURE MIX

Combine all the Acupressure techniques into a thorough massage of the entire eye region. Do a few seconds of Acupressure A, then a few seconds of Acupressure B, then a few seconds of Acupressure C. Massage the entire rim of the eye socket and surrounding area until your eyes feel pleasantly invigorated and refreshed. You can increase the amount of stimulation by tapping the skin with the tips of your fingers several times a second. Use two or three fingers together for a more powerful effect.

TECHNIQUE #13: LIGHT THERAPY

Sit about 6 inches away from a strong bright light, preferably 150 watt, with your eyes closed and relaxed. The light should make your eyes feel pleasantly warm but not too hot. If you're unduly sensitive to light, sit as close as possible and reduce the distance to 6 inches as the discomfort subsides. Within a few days you should be desensitized. Gently swing your head from side to side so that each eye receives an equal amount of light.

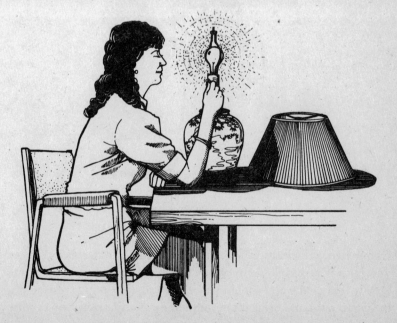

As you bathe your closed eyes in the light, repeat your affirmation and visualize the inner lens becoming more flexible and the ciliary muscle becoming more powerful. Visualize the extraocular muscles massaging the eyeball and making it healthier. It doesn't matter if you get clear images or cartoon characters. The important thing is to couple the affirmation with vivid images of your eyes changing for the better. This technique will leave your eyes feeling wonderfully refreshed.

TECHNIQUE #14: PALMING

Close your eyes and cover them with your hands so that no light gets in. Rest the heel of your palms on your cheekbones and cross your hands on your forehead. Don't press against your eyeballs and make sure your eyelids, eyebrows, and the rest of the eye region is relaxed. Repeat your affirmation and visualize positive changes taking place inside your eyes, just as with Light Therapy.

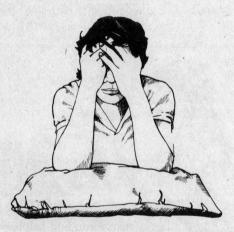

TECHNIQUE #15: HYDROTHERAPY

Obtain two washcloths, a bowl of hot water, and a bowl of cold water. The hot water should be very hot but not so hot that it scalds the eyelids. The cold water should be ice cold, so keep a bowl of water in the refrigerator and bring it out for therapy. Alternatively, you can use an ice pack. Now dip a washcloth in the hot water and hold it against your closed eyes for thirty seconds. Now do the same thing with the cold washcloth. Continue to alternate hot and cold washcloths while repeating your affirmation and visualizing positive changes inside your eyes. Finish by gently massaging your closed eyes with a dry towel.

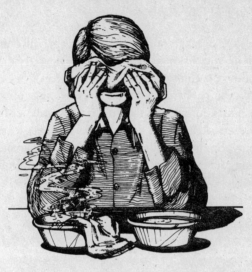

TECHNIQUE #16: AVERSION THERAPY

If you hate your glasses, you'll love this technique. Studies of cancer patients have shown that spontaneous remission occurs most often in patients who curse and revile the tumors. A similar technique can be used in the fight against poor vision.

Many people who wear glasses carry deep emotional scars. Feelings of inferiority, disappointment, frustration, and helplessness are common among spectacle wearers. The adage *"Guys don't make passes at girls who wear glasses"* has undoubtedly caused many tears to flow from tender teenage eyes. These emotional wounds must be healed. The best way of doing this is through aversion therapy.

When you've adapted to a weaker prescription, the previous pair of glasses will be too strong. Don't just throw them away. Smash them up!

Take a hammer or put on your stomping boots and vent all those pent-up negative emotions. With every blow, release those feelings of anger, frustration, and helplessness. Get the adrenaline flowing and work up a sweat. Get the negativity out of your system. Don't be inhibited. Shout and curse and scream and make the act of destruction a powerful symbol of your commitment to better vision!

As you release these emotions you may experience an *immediate* improvement in your vision as you release the negativity. Just let yourself go and allow the emotions to flow. A few words of caution. Make sure you really can see better with the weaker prescription. You don't want to smash up your glasses, then realize you still need them. If you can use the frames, keep them. Poke out the stronger lenses with your thumbs. Then wrap them in adhesive tape and put them in plastic bags before smashing them up so shards of glass don't fly about.

6

TEN SIMPLE STRATEGIES

HOW TO GET FASTER RESULTS

Before giving you the Strategies and Booster Sequences, we have some advice on how to set things up so that you get really fast results. Do everything as directed and don't take shortcuts or skip anything. Once you've mastered the techniques you can unleash your creativity. Until then, do things our way and learn the method correctly. This chapter contains a lot of important information, so study it carefully. If you need stress-relieving glasses or a weaker prescription, show your eye doctor the prescribing guidelines in the Appendix.

- *Rearrange your schedule.* Most people spend several hours a day watching TV. If you just reduce your TV viewing by ½ hour a day for one month, you'll have plenty of time. Simply rearrange your priorities and carefully cultivate the habit of doing the Booster Sequences every day. Once they become habitual, you'll actually look forward to them because they'll make you feel good. They'll make you feel energized, relaxed, and positive about yourself.

- *Use an alarm clock.* Since habits thrive on regularity, you should do the Booster Sequences at the same time every day. The best way to remind yourself is to use an alarm clock. This is easily the most powerful technique available for developing new habits. Don't risk failure by relying on memory because you'll probably get sidetracked and forget. Use an alarm clock. When doing the therapy, unplug the phone, switch off the TV, and don't let anything distract you.

• *Read every chapter several times.* Become thoroughly familiar with the material. Don't be discouraged if you don't understand everything at first. Most of the information will be new to you and will take time to sink in. So don't get discouraged. Just read each chapter several times and everything will become perfectly clear.

• *Set up a special place.* Find a spot that has good lighting and about 6 feet of blank wall. Objects in the background will give you annoying double images when doing Tromboning. You'll also need a table and chair for Light Therapy, Palming, and Hydrotherapy. Attach the charts to the wall or a piece of card to hold in your hand. Leave everything in place to remind you to do the therapy.

• *Obtain a 150-watt lightbulb for light therapy.* Although 100 watts is OK, 150 watts is better and is worth the trip to the store.

• *Photocopy the Booster Sequences.* These are given later in this chapter. Use a fresh copy every week and check the boxes as you do the techniques. Aim for a perfect week with at least one Booster Sequence per day. Each Booster Sequence is thirty minutes. Don't let a day go by without doing some vision therapy. If you miss a day, do an extra Booster Sequence the next day or on the weekend.

• *Do the booster sequences to music unless you prefer silence.* Put on background music and/or use a kitchen timer. Special cassette tapes are available from AVI; mail the Response Form at the back of the book. Try to do the Booster Sequences without "corrective" lenses or use a weaker prescription. Experiment and see what works best for you. If your goal is just to stabilize your vision at its present level, wear your current prescription.

• *Keep a journal and record your progress.* Once a week, measure the distance from the bridge of your nose to your blur zone. Also make a note of the smallest line you can see on the Acuity Chart at 14 inches and at 10 feet. The best time for these measurements is early in the day, when your eyes are fresh and relaxed. Record how much time you spend without "corrective" lenses and other changes in your vision. Keeping a record is important because it's a powerful motivating force. For example, if you're myopic and your blur zone is 18 inches away when you start the therapy and 26 inches away by the end of the second week, you'll know for a fact that your vision is improving and that you're really getting results.

- *Upgrade your diet.* Avoid junk food, especially sugar, because it can make the inner lens swell up and aggravate myopia. Poor diet can also increase the risk of cataract and macular degeneration. Instead, follow these guidelines. Eat less fat. Drink plenty of liquids. Eat whole-grain cereals. Don't add salt to your food. Eat lots of fruits and vegetables. Take a multivitamin supplement.

- *Reward yourself.* After every Booster Sequence, do something enjoyable, like eating some fruit or a small piece of chocolate.

- *Verbally motivate yourself.* Repeat your affirmation often and give yourself pep talks to stay motivated and activate your body's natural healing process. Verbally remind yourself of the improvement in your vision.

- *Wear sunglasses outdoors during the daytime.* It's important to stop ultraviolet light from entering the eyes because it's a major cause of cataract and macular degeneration. Get the lightest tint available so that your pupil doesn't dilate and make sure the tag states that they actually block ultraviolet light.

- *Wear an eyepatch.* Get one from your local drugstore and wear it for an hour or more a day when reading, watching TV, or playing. Don't wear it for potentially dangerous activities such as cooking, using power tools, crossing the road, or driving. An eyepatch is one of the best vision therapy techniques available because it forces each eye to work and will really accelerate your progress. If you have a lazy eye, wear it longer over the dominant eye so that the lazy eye gets plenty of work.

- *Don't skip hydrotherapy or the eyepatch.* Some people can't be bothered with these techniques and may fail to get results. Hydrotherapy is one of the best things you can do for your eyes because it stimulates the flow of nutrients. An eyepatch is also a very powerful technique and you must resist the temptation to avoid or remove it. It doesn't take up any extra time because you'll be wearing it for things that you do anyway. So discipline yourself and wear it until you get used to it!

- *Don't be lazy.* Remember that your eyes must last a lifetime and that it only takes a month to master our method. So make this Vision Therapy Month and learn the techniques. Don't be impatient if your vision doesn't improve as fast as you want and don't try to force your eyes to see better. Just cultivate the habit of doing the therapy every day and your vision will improve of its own accord.

- *Use the potentiation effect.* When you've mastered the techniques, try doing them for longer periods of time. For example, fifteen minutes of continuous Pumping gives better results than five separate periods of three minutes. This is known as the *potentiation effect.*

- *Release your creativity.* At the end of a month, you'll have a good idea of which techniques are working best for you and can even create your own Booster Sequences to emphasize the most effective techniques. Of course, you can continue to use the Booster Sequences in this book.

ADVICE FOR COMPUTER USERS

Modify your work routine to prevent stress from building up. The best way is to do a Slow Blink every few minutes. *Set yourself the goal of doing at least 100 Slow Blinks per day.* Don't just rely on memory, or you'll probably get sidetracked and forget. It's much better to keep a written record using bars and gates. Every time you do a Slow Blink, look at a distant object, then add another bar to the gate. This simple technique is highly recommended because it can rapidly reduce computer eyestrain and headaches.

~~||||~~ ~~||||~~~~||||~~ ~~||||~~ ~~||||~~~~||||~~ ~~||||~~~~||||~~ |||

Computer users should get up, stretch, and walk around every 30 minutes. The law entitles you to a five-minute alternate work break every thirty minutes, so take advantage of it. Also, whenever the computer is busy processing something and you're waiting for it to finish, look at a distant object. Another good idea is to program your screen saver to remind you to do a Slow Blink or look at a distant object every few minutes.

STUDY YOUR BLUR ZONE

Most people have a zone of clear vision and a blur zone where everything is blurred. If you have a lot of astigmatism, hyperopia, or presbyopia, things may be blurred at all distances. The AVI Program will increase your clear zone and decrease your blur zone. Simply by developing the habit of carefully studying blurred objects, your blur zone will start to clear up and you'll experience a major improvement in your vision.

When doing Blur Zoning as part of a Booster Sequence, put an interesting object with lots of detail partly into your blur zone so that some of it is clear but most of it is blurred. Slowly run your gaze along the edges for a few seconds, then carefully study the *smallest details* you can see. For example, if you're using a plant, follow the outlines of the leaves, then study small details such as tiny veins or pores in the surface. Aim for calm, relaxed, contemplative vision without squinting or any other tricks.

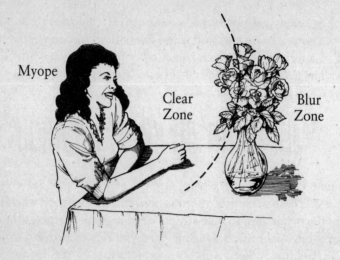

NOW FOR THE STRATEGIES

This section is comprehensive, but not as complicated as it looks. Study it carefully and select the Booster Sequence for your visual problem. If you have a cluster of visual problems, alternate the Booster Sequences for each problem. For example, if you're myopic and the aging process is also affecting you, do the Myopia Booster Sequence one day and the Presbyopia Booster Sequence the next.

1. VISION THERAPY FOR EYESTRAIN

It's essential to minimize stress, especially visual stress, because it can seriously degrade the performance of the visual system. The following symptoms often occur after long periods of reading or computer work and usually respond to vision therapy and/or stress-relieving glasses.

- *Tics and tension in eyelids*
- *Headache, jitters, indigestion*
- *Dry, tired, aching, bloodshot eyes*

- *Loss of concentration and accuracy*
- *Fatigue, anxiety, irritability, insomnia*
- *Blurred or double vision, even with glasses*
- *Clumsy, accident prone, bumping into things*

If you suffer from any of these symptoms, do the Stress-Reduction Booster Sequences first. When the discomfort subsides, do whatever Booster Sequences are appropriate for your visual problem. For example, if you're myopic and are suffering from eyestrain, do the Stress-Reduction Booster Sequences for a few days, then do the Myopia Booster Sequences when your eyes are feeling better.

STRESS-REDUCTION BOOSTER SEQUENCE 1

Light Therapy	7 minutes	☐	☐	☐	☐	☐	☐	☐
Palming	7 minutes	☐	☐	☐	☐	☐	☐	☐
Light Therapy	7 minutes	☐	☐	☐	☐	☐	☐	☐
Palming	7 minutes	☐	☐	☐	☐	☐	☐	☐

STRESS-REDUCTION BOOSTER SEQUENCE 2

Hydrotherapy	5 minutes	☐	☐	☐	☐	☐	☐	☐
Acupressure Mix	5 minutes	☐	☐	☐	☐	☐	☐	☐
Light Therapy	10 minutes	☐	☐	☐	☐	☐	☐	☐
Palming	10 minutes	☐	☐	☐	☐	☐	☐	☐

2. VISION THERAPY FOR PROGRESSIVE MYOPIA

This section is for myopes who are getting progressively worse and periodically need stronger prescriptions. There are different strategies for different amounts of myopia:

- If you can read or do computer work without "corrective" lenses, stop wearing them for these activities. Reading through "corrective" lenses is the major cause of progressive myopia, so stop wearing them for close work. Most people who use this strategy become free from glasses most of the time and need them only for driving and other activities that require good distance vision. This strategy works best for people with less than 3.00D of myopia, although many people with larger amounts of myopia use it successfully.

- If you have a small amount of myopia and can use stress-relieving glasses, these will help reverse the myopia and return you to normal vision. This strategy works best for people with less than 1.50D of myopia.

- If you can't read without "corrective lenses," use the weakest pair that you can get by with. The goal is to wear glasses that give you clear vision at your usual reading distance but make everything further away blurred. Many people have old weaker glasses that will suffice. If not, ask your eye doctor to prescribe weaker glasses for reading. Many people find that as their myopia improves they can use the weaker glasses for distance vision.

- If your work requires you to look up frequently and see distant objects clearly, you should use Professor Young's formula. These are bifocals with weaker distance lenses at the top coupled with stress-relieving lenses at the bottom. The complete formula is given in the Appendix and is especially useful for schoolchildren.

- If you wear contact lenses, you have several options. Hard contact lenses and some gas permeable lenses can stop or slow down progressive myopia. If you are interested in trying these lenses, consult a contact lens specialist and ask him what his success rate is.

- You can remove your contact lenses for reading so you reduce nearpoint stress. Depending on the severity of your myopia, you may be able to wear just one contact lens. Use the eye with the contact lens for distance vision and the eye without the contact lens for reading. Another option is to wear stress-relieving glasses over your contact lenses.

PROGRESSIVE MYOPIA BOOSTER SEQUENCE 1

Hydrotherapy	3 minutes	☐	☐	☐	☐	☐	☐	☐
Fast Blinking	1 minute	☐	☐	☐	☐	☐	☐	☐
Slow Blinking	1 minute	☐	☐	☐	☐	☐	☐	☐
Squeeze Blinking	1 minute	☐	☐	☐	☐	☐	☐	☐
Pumping	3 minutes	☐	☐	☐	☐	☐	☐	☐
Eye Rolls	1 minute	☐	☐	☐	☐	☐	☐	☐
Clock Rotations	1 minute	☐	☐	☐	☐	☐	☐	☐
Pumping	3 minutes	☐	☐	☐	☐	☐	☐	☐
Light Therapy	5 minutes	☐	☐	☐	☐	☐	☐	☐
Acupressure A	2 minutes	☐	☐	☐	☐	☐	☐	☐
Acupressure B	2 minutes	☐	☐	☐	☐	☐	☐	☐
Acupressure C	2 minutes	☐	☐	☐	☐	☐	☐	☐
Palming	5 minutes	☐	☐	☐	☐	☐	☐	☐

PROGRESSIVE MYOPIA BOOSTER SEQUENCE 2

Hydrotherapy	3 minutes	☐	☐	☐	☐	☐	☐	☐
Pumping	3 minutes	☐	☐	☐	☐	☐	☐	☐
Acuity Chart	2 minutes	☐	☐	☐	☐	☐	☐	☐
Scanning Chart	2 minutes	☐	☐	☐	☐	☐	☐	☐
Pumping	3 minutes	☐	☐	☐	☐	☐	☐	☐
Blur Zoning	2 minutes	☐	☐	☐	☐	☐	☐	☐
Acupressure Mix	5 minutes	☐	☐	☐	☐	☐	☐	☐
Light Therapy	5 minutes	☐	☐	☐	☐	☐	☐	☐
Palming	5 minutes	☐	☐	☐	☐	☐	☐	☐

Another New Visual Habit: Seeing Space

A common problem for myopes is that they spend so much time reading or focusing on the computer screen that their peripheral vision literally fades away and they end up with tunnel vision. To correct this problem, add the following technique to your New Visual Habits. It's called *Seeing Space* and can often produce major improvements in vision.

Look at a distant object but don't pay any attention to it. Breathe slowly and deeply and relax. Try to enter into a detached, dreamy state of mind and notice all the things around you using your peripheral vision. Take in as much space as possible and look for smaller and smaller details using your peripheral vision, down to the limits of your perception. Use this technique at traffic lights, at your workstation, and during TV commercials.

You should also develop the habit of using your central vision to carefully study the most distant objects you can see, with or without "corrective" lenses. For example, at traffic lights look at objects a mile away. The goal is to regain full awareness of space with both central and peripheral vision.

3. VISION THERAPY FOR STABLE MYOPIA

The techniques given above will usually stabilize progressive myopia within a few weeks. When you can see that your vision is improving, or you're already stable and didn't need a stronger prescription when you had your last eye exam, you're ready for the next step. If you didn't already do so, read the section on progressive myopia before proceeding.

- Whether you wear glasses or contact lenses, concentrate on adapting to weaker prescriptions. Use old weaker glasses or contact lenses from previous years or ask your eye doctor for a weaker prescription.

STABLE MYOPIA BOOSTER SEQUENCE 1

Hydrotherapy	3 minutes	☐	☐	☐	☐	☐	☐	☐
Fusion Chart	2 minutes	☐	☐	☐	☐	☐	☐	☐
Pumping	3 minutes	☐	☐	☐	☐	☐	☐	☐
Blur Zoning	2 minutes	☐	☐	☐	☐	☐	☐	☐
Acupressure Mix	5 minutes	☐	☐	☐	☐	☐	☐	☐
Squeeze Blinking	2 minutes	☐	☐	☐	☐	☐	☐	☐
Pumping	3 minutes	☐	☐	☐	☐	☐	☐	☐
Light Therapy	5 minutes	☐	☐	☐	☐	☐	☐	☐
Palming	5 minutes	☐	☐	☐	☐	☐	☐	☐

STABLE MYOPIA BOOSTER SEQUENCE 2

Hydrotherapy	3 minutes	☐	☐	☐	☐	☐	☐	☐
Fusion Pumping	3 minutes	☐	☐	☐	☐	☐	☐	☐
Squeeze Blinking	2 minutes	☐	☐	☐	☐	☐	☐	☐
Clock Rotations	2 minutes	☐	☐	☐	☐	☐	☐	☐
Fusion Pumping	3 minutes	☐	☐	☐	☐	☐	☐	☐
Eye Rolls	2 minutes	☐	☐	☐	☐	☐	☐	☐
Clock Rotations	2 minutes	☐	☐	☐	☐	☐	☐	☐
Fusion Pumping	3 minutes	☐	☐	☐	☐	☐	☐	☐
Light Therapy	5 minutes	☐	☐	☐	☐	☐	☐	☐
Palming	5 minutes	☐	☐	☐	☐	☐	☐	☐

• If you wear contact lenses, try disposables. These will enable you to adapt to weaker prescriptions every few weeks without spending a ton of money. Ask your eye doctor for an entire series of progressively weaker lenses so that you can reduce the strength as needed. If your myopia is not too bad, you may be able to wear one contact lens for distance vision and nothing in the other eye for reading.

Some final words of advice. Instead of compulsively reading page after page without stopping, discipline yourself to use the Bookmark for all your major reading. This is really important. You must break the habit of constantly focusing on close objects! Take regular vision therapy breaks and gaze at distant objects. Spend more time outdoors. Play vision improving games such as Frisbee, golf, tennis, and bowling.

There's one more technique that you should use on a daily basis. Although not suitable for the Booster Sequences, this technique can rapidly improve your vision by teaching you how to bring blurred objects into focus and is well worth the extra few minutes. Please give it a try. You'll be surprised how effective it is.

Supplementary Technique A: Candle Power

Put a candle or small light bulb at the other end of a dark room. If you use a candle, make sure there are no drafts because you want a steady flame. Now cover one eye with an eyepatch and gaze at the light, which will be blurred. Breathe slowly and deeply and try to make the image as small as possible. By paying close attention to the sensation inside your eyes, you'll learn how to consciously control your ciliary muscle and make the inner lens thinner. Do this for five minutes with one eye covered, then cover the other eye and repeat the procedure. Don't use "corrective" lenses. When you can do this technique easily with an eyepatch, practice making blurred objects clearer using both eyes together during your normal daily activities. Your goal is to look at blurred objects and bring them into focus simply by pulling on your ciliary muscles.

4. Vision Therapy for Astigmatism

Most people with astigmatism have bad posture, with the head habitually tilted to one side. To correct this problem, tilt your head an equal amount in the opposite direction. This causes the extraocular muscles to adjust the force they exert on the eyeball as they adapt to the new head position, which helps neutralize the astigmatism.

ASTIGMATISM BOOSTER SEQUENCE

Hydrotherapy	3 minutes	☐	☐	☐	☐	☐	☐ ☐
Eye Rolls	1 minute	☐	☐	☐	☐	☐	☐ ☐
Clock Rotations	1 minute	☐	☐	☐	☐	☐	☐ ☐
Acupressure A	2 minutes	☐	☐	☐	☐	☐	☐ ☐
Eye Rolls	1 minute	☐	☐	☐	☐	☐	☐ ☐
Clock Rotations	1 minute	☐	☐	☐	☐	☐	☐ ☐
Acupressure B	2 minutes	☐	☐	☐	☐	☐	☐ ☐
Eye Rolls	1 minute	☐	☐	☐	☐	☐	☐ ☐
Clock Rotations	1 minute	☐	☐	☐	☐	☐	☐ ☐
Acupressure C	2 minutes	☐	☐	☐	☐	☐	☐ ☐
Fast Blinking	1 minute	☐	☐	☐	☐	☐	☐ ☐
Slow Blinking	1 minute	☐	☐	☐	☐	☐	☐ ☐
Squeeze Blinking	1 minute	☐	☐	☐	☐	☐	☐ ☐
Acuity Chart	2 minutes	☐	☐	☐	☐	☐	☐ ☐
Light Therapy	5 minutes	☐	☐	☐	☐	☐	☐ ☐
Palming	5 minutes	☐	☐	☐	☐	☐	☐ ☐

Stand in front of a mirror and notice which way your head habitually tilts. Ask a friend to give you a second opinion. Then make some cards to remind yourself to tilt your head the opposite way. For example, if you habitually tilt your head 25 degrees to the left, tilt it 25 degrees to the right for the next few months.

Put a dozen cards in prominent places around the house, in your car, and at work. Whenever you look at a card, make sure your head is tilted in the new direction and stretch your neck muscles. This will feel strange, but you'll soon get used to it. The Astigmatism Booster Sequence may make your eyes rather sore. If so, substitute the Stress-Reduction Booster Sequences for a few days.

5. Vision Therapy for Presbyopia and Hyperopia

As we get older, the inner lens loses flexibility and focusing power. This can cause serious complications because the inner lens doesn't contain any blood vessels and absorbs nutrients from the surrounding liquid and eliminates toxic waste products by means of diffusion. When the inner lens changes focus, it facilitates this process and engages in a type of "breathing" action. In contrast, when the inner lens becomes stiff, it stops "breathing." Nutrients can't enter as easily and toxic waste products build up, clogging the tiny channels inside the lens and increasing the risk of cataract. Similar problems affect the retina and increase the risk of macular degeneration.

Hence vision therapy for presbyopia is mostly concerned with stimulating activity in the entire eye region. The goal is to maximize the flexibility of the inner lens and increase the nutrient flow. This makes the eye healthier and helps it continue functioning efficiently. The major symptom of presbyopia is loss of close focusing power, hence the Presbyopia Booster Sequences are also suitable for hyperopia.

If you can read without "corrective" lenses, don't use them. If you can't read without them, use the weakest pair possible. If you have a small amount of astigmatism, drugstore reading glasses are almost as good as prescription glasses. If you wear bifocals or trifocals, try to

PRESBYOPIA (HYPEROPIA) BOOSTER SEQUENCE 1

Hydrotherapy	3 minutes	☐	☐	☐	☐	☐	☐	☐
Fast Blinking	1 minute	☐	☐	☐	☐	☐	☐	☐
Slow Blinking	1 minute	☐	☐	☐	☐	☐	☐	☐
Squeeze Blinking	1 minute	☐	☐	☐	☐	☐	☐	☐
Pumping	3 minutes	☐	☐	☐	☐	☐	☐	☐
Nose Fusion	1 minute	☐	☐	☐	☐	☐	☐	☐
Eye Rolls	1 minute	☐	☐	☐	☐	☐	☐	☐
Clock Rotations	1 minute	☐	☐	☐	☐	☐	☐	☐
Tromboning	3 minutes	☐	☐	☐	☐	☐	☐	☐
Nose Fusion	1 minute	☐	☐	☐	☐	☐	☐	☐
Fusion Chart	2 minutes	☐	☐	☐	☐	☐	☐	☐
Blur Zoning	2 minutes	☐	☐	☐	☐	☐	☐	☐
Light Therapy	5 minutes	☐	☐	☐	☐	☐	☐	☐
Palming	5 minutes	☐	☐	☐	☐	☐	☐	☐

return to single-vision lenses. If you wear contact lenses, you may be able to wear one contact lens for reading and nothing in the other eye, which you'll use for distance vision.

6. VISION THERAPY FOR LAZY AND CROSSED EYES

Even though many ophthalmologists still use surgery for crossed eyes, this method is basically obsolete and shouldn't be considered unless other options have failed. Vision therapy and a drug known as *Oculinum* are much more effective. Oculinum is the commercial name for botulinum toxin, which paralyzes muscles for about six weeks. The drug is injected into the extraocular muscles to straighten the eyes. The

PRESBYOPIA (HYPEROPIA) BOOSTER SEQUENCE 2

Hydrotherapy	3 minutes	☐	☐	☐	☐	☐	☐	☐
Eye Rolls	1 minute	☐	☐	☐	☐	☐	☐	☐
Clock Rotations	1 minute	☐	☐	☐	☐	☐	☐	☐
Acupressure Mix	3 minutes	☐	☐	☐	☐	☐	☐	☐
Blur Reading	2 minutes	☐	☐	☐	☐	☐	☐	☐
Pumping	3 minutes	☐	☐	☐	☐	☐	☐	☐
Acuity Chart	2 minutes	☐	☐	☐	☐	☐	☐	☐
Scanning Chart	2 minutes	☐	☐	☐	☐	☐	☐	☐
Tromboning	3 minutes	☐	☐	☐	☐	☐	☐	☐
Light Therapy	5 minutes	☐	☐	☐	☐	☐	☐	☐
Palming	5 minutes	☐	☐	☐	☐	☐	☐	☐

eyes usually remain straight when the drug eventually wears off. Of course, vision therapy should also be used to make both eyes work together as a team.

An effective technique for amblyopia and strabismus is to wear an eyepatch several hours a day to force the weaker eye to develop. Once the weaker eye is working better, use the Myopia Booster Sequences and the Presbyopia Booster Sequences to improve eye movements and coordination. Many behavioral optometrists offer more advanced techniques and have a very high success rate.

7. VISION THERAPY FOR DRY EYE SYNDROME

Many contact lens wearers and older people suffer from dry eyes, because their tear glands malfunction and don't produce enough tear fluid or produce tear fluid of the wrong composition. Your New Visual Habits should emphasize Slow Blinking and Squeeze Blinking to stimulate the production of tear fluid.

DRY EYE SYNDROME BOOSTER SEQUENCE

Hydrotherapy	3 minutes	☐	☐	☐	☐	☐	☐	☐
Acupressure A	2 minutes	☐	☐	☐	☐	☐	☐	☐
Slow Blinking	2 minutes	☐	☐	☐	☐	☐	☐	☐
Squeeze Blinking	2 minutes	☐	☐	☐	☐	☐	☐	☐
Acupressure B	2 minutes	☐	☐	☐	☐	☐	☐	☐
Slow Blinking	2 minutes	☐	☐	☐	☐	☐	☐	☐
Squeeze Blinking	2 minutes	☐	☐	☐	☐	☐	☐	☐
Acupressure C	2 minutes	☐	☐	☐	☐	☐	☐	☐
Light Therapy	5 minutes	☐	☐	☐	☐	☐	☐	☐
Palming	5 minutes	☐	☐	☐	☐	☐	☐	☐
Acupressure Mix	3 minutes	☐	☐	☐	☐	☐	☐	☐

8. VISION THERAPY FOR YOUNG CHILDREN

During the first few months of life, a baby should have plenty of bright, moving objects to look at so that it learns how to use its eyes properly. Put the crib away from a wall and hang colored toys above its head. Don't let young children watch TV less than 10 feet away. When the child can read, it should be taught the New Visual Habits described in Chapter 4 to prevent visual problems. If glasses are needed for any reason, the child should not be made to wear them full-time because they will stop the eyes from developing normally.

9. VISION THERAPY FOR CATARACT

The eye's inner lens consists of billions of living cells. When these die, they form a cataract, which is simply the accumulation of cellular debris. Major causes of cataract include low nutrient levels, ultraviolet light, and toxic waste products. Cataracts are not contagious and are sometimes reversible.

The basic strategy for cataract therapy is to boost nutrient levels and stimulate activity in the inner lens to restore its "breathing" action. The goal is to revitalize the cells and flush out toxic waste products and cellular debris, which makes the inner lens more transparent. Clinical experience suggests that cataracts can often be significantly improved within three months, eliminating or delaying the need for surgery.

In addition to a strong multivitamin supplement, we recommend taking the following quantities of extra nutrients every day: 50 mg of zinc; 400 units of vitamin E; 10,000 units of beta-carotene; and a vitamin B complex. The important thing is to provide the eyes with high levels of these nutrients so that they can work their way into the lens and reverse the damage. You should also do the following Booster Sequence twice a day:

CATARACT BOOSTER SEQUENCE

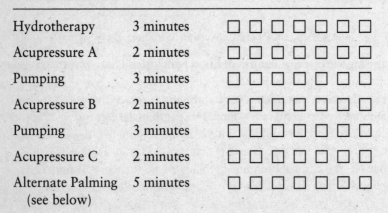

Hydrotherapy	3 minutes	☐ ☐ ☐ ☐ ☐ ☐ ☐
Acupressure A	2 minutes	☐ ☐ ☐ ☐ ☐ ☐ ☐
Pumping	3 minutes	☐ ☐ ☐ ☐ ☐ ☐ ☐
Acupressure B	2 minutes	☐ ☐ ☐ ☐ ☐ ☐ ☐
Pumping	3 minutes	☐ ☐ ☐ ☐ ☐ ☐ ☐
Acupressure C	2 minutes	☐ ☐ ☐ ☐ ☐ ☐ ☐
Alternate Palming (see below)	5 minutes	☐ ☐ ☐ ☐ ☐ ☐ ☐

Supplementary Technique B: Alternate Palming

Sit about 9 inches in front of a 150-watt lightbulb with your eyes closed, as for Light Therapy. Cover your eyes with your hands for fifteen seconds, as in normal Palming, and let your eyes adapt to the darkness. Then remove your hands and bathe your *closed* eyes in the light for fifteen seconds. Now cover your eyes again and have fifteen more seconds of darkness. Continue to alternate fifteen seconds of light and fifteen seconds of darkness, keeping your eyes closed at all times. This important technique improves the circulation of fluids inside the eye, especially around the inner lens.

10. VISION THERAPY FOR MACULAR DEGENERATION

Finally, a few words about macular degeneration, which is caused in much the same way as cataract. The cells at the back of the retina die and debris known as *drusen* accumulates. Vision therapy often yields improvement but not a cure. The nutrients and therapy techniques are the same as for cataract therapy. We also recommend taking 60 mg of bilberry herbal extract per day, plus 5,000 mg of vitamin C and 500 mg of taurine (an amino acid). These supplements should be taken with food to avoid stomach irritation.

GENERAL SIGNS OF PROGRESS

Regardless of your visual problem, your range of clear vision should increase. If you're myopic, your blur zone should move away from you and distant objects will become clearer. If you're hyperopic or presbyopic, your blur zone should move toward you and near objects will become clearer. If you have astigmatism, objects at all distances should become clearer. If you're using a weaker prescription, you should be able to see more clearly through it. If you're stabilizing your vision, you should be able to see more clearly through your current prescription.

Cultivate the habit of doing some vision therapy every day and establish a routine you can live with, just as you habitually brush your hair and clean your teeth every day. For example, when you're learning the Booster Sequences, you may find it more convenient to do fifteen minutes in the morning and fifteen minutes in the evening. Once you've mastered the method, you can probably cut back to ten minutes a day or just do vision therapy at traffic lights. Experiment and find the right way of fitting the therapy into your lifestyle.

Whatever it takes, don't let bad thoughts and feelings stop you from doing the therapy! If you make yourself do the Booster Sequences, the negativity will quickly evaporate, leaving you energized, confident, and relaxed. If you feel tense and uptight, do some vision therapy! If you feel gloomy and depressed, do some vision therapy! If you feel lazy and lethargic, do some vision therapy! *Resolutely do it even if you don't feel like doing it because it will make you feel better. You'll be glad you did!*

YOU CAN MAKE A DIFFERENCE

LAY DOWN YOUR SILVER

The origin of "corrective" lenses dates back to 1286 A.D., when the medieval scholar Roger Bacon discovered that a magnifying glass helped him read more easily. A few years later, the Italian craftsmen Alexander de Spina and Salvina D'Amati attached magnifying lenses to wire frames and invented the first spectacles. Long before the advent of the eye examination, spectacles were sold in marketplaces by jewelers, hatters, tinkers, and tailors. A poem by John Lydgate (1370–1450) is the first known reference to spectacle vending:

> Master, what will you buy? Fine felt hats, or spectacles
> to read? Lay down your silver and here you may speed.

Just as modern drugstores sell reading glasses from display racks, the early spectacle vendors offered a selection that browsing customers could try on and choose to their liking. Jewelers dominated the market because their expertise in metal working enabled them to make superior frames and many of them set up proprietary schools.

The end of the nineteenth century saw the birth of optometry. Advances in optical science allowed spectacle vendors to perform eye examinations and a new class of practitioners emerged who called themselves *refracting opticians*. Their techniques made spectacle selection more precise, and they decided to form a new profession, just as dentists and physicians were doing.

Working hand-in-glove with the optical glass industry, the refracting opticians founded the American Optometric Association in 1904, coining the term *Doctor of Optometry* to describe themselves. Because physicians also treated eyes, they formed their own branch of the eye care profession, known as *ophthalmology*.

THE FACADE OF PROFESSIONAL UNITY

During the next few decades, intense legal conflicts took place in every state as the American Optometric Association battled the American Medical Association over treatment procedures and financial territory. These conflicts continue to the present day through academic journals, advertising campaigns, legislation, and the courts, as large numbers of eye doctors fight each other for patients and health care dollars.

The eye care establishment tries to downplay these conflicts and wants the public to think that eye doctors are a big happy family, marching forward together along the path of progress and selflessly serving their patients. This is totally misleading. Bitter rivalry between the different factions has seriously impeded the flow of information regarding some major advances, especially in behavioral optometry.

The truth is that important research findings are routinely ignored or suppressed by those traditional eye doctors whose only concern is to preserve the status quo. In many cases, the desire of traditional eye doctors to maintain their high income levels has won out over the best interest of their patients, who are deliberately misled or not given enough information to make intelligent decisions. Fortunately, a growing number of health-conscious individuals have penetrated the facade and are turning things around.

The explosive growth of alternative health care is more than just a fad. It reflects a widespread dissatisfaction with the status quo. Large numbers of people are fed up with the same old answers. They realize that health problems don't just fall out of the sky and hit them on the head, and they're tired of being given the runaround by doctors who try to belittle them and downplay their concerns. That is why we're providing you with enough information to make an intelligent decision about the way your eyes should be treated.

CONCERNED DOCTORS SPEAK OUT

The basic problem with "corrective" lenses is that they don't really correct anything. Think about it: if they did, people would wear them for a while, and then wouldn't need them anymore because their eyes would have returned to normal. A vast amount of clinical experience, as well as countless complaints from patients leave no doubt that "corrective" lenses usually create dependency and make the eyes lose even more of their natural focusing power. Professor Young explains:

The worst thing you can do for myopia is to treat it with "corrective" lenses. These increase the level of accommodation when used for close work and cause further deterioration. If treated with bifocals or vision therapy, myopia should be a transitory condition like a headache that eventually goes away. Instead, "corrective" lenses aggravate the problem and condemn the patient to a lifetime of dependency.

Over the years, many other doctors have voiced their concerns:

Full correction for distance vision causes the myope to produce extra accommodation when viewing close objects with their lenses on. Since excessive accommodation is implicated in the etiology of myopia, the eye may become more myopic when fully corrected.
J. Angle and D. A. Wissman, *Soc. Sci. Med.*, 14A: 473–479, 1980.

Single-vision minus lenses for full-time use produce accommoda-tive insufficiency associated with additional symptoms until the patient gets used to the lenses. This is usually accompanied by a further increase in myopia and the cycle begins anew.
M. H. Birnbaum, *Rev. Optom.*, 110(21): 23–29, 1973.

The emphasis on compensatory lenses has posed a problem for many years in our examinations. These lenses do not correct anything and may not serve the patient in his best interest over a period of time.
C. J. Forkiotis, *OEP*, 53:1, 1980.

Spectacle lenses can create their own problems. There are fre-quently ignored patterns of addiction to minus lenses. The typical prescription tends to overpower and fatigue the visual system and what is often a transient condition becomes a lifelong situation, which is likely to deteriorate with time.
S. Gallop, *J. Behav. Optom.*, 5(5): 115–120, 1994.

The use of compensatory lenses to treat or neutralize the symp-toms does not correct or cure the problem. The current education and training of eye care practitioners discourages preventive and remedial treatment.
R. L. Gottlieb, *J. Optom. Vis. Dev.*, 13(1): 3–27, 1982.

I have yet to hear of a research paper confirming the beneficial effects of prescribing compensatory lenses. I'm sure most optom-etrists will confirm the clinical observation that patients who re-ceive compensatory lenses for full time wear are usually the ones who need a stronger prescription every year.
J. Liberman, *J. Am. Optom. Assoc.*, 47(8): 1058–1064, 1976.

Concave lenses are the most common approach, yet the least likely to prevent further myopic progression. Unfortunately, they increase the nearpoint stress that is associated with pro-gression.
B. May, *OEP*, A-112, 1984.

THE EMPEROR HAS NO CLOTHES

Although almost 100,000 research papers have been published on the eyes, some vitally important topics seem to be "off limits" and have never been investigated. These involve the effects of "corrective" lenses on the ciliary muscle and inner lens. Merely to say that large gaps exist in our knowledge is an understatement. Almost nothing is known about these products except that they often cause dependency and deterioration.

The truth is that no clinical studies have ever demonstrated the long-term safety or effectiveness of "corrective" lenses. *To put it bluntly, the traditional method of prescribing these products is an untested and unproven form of treatment.* In fact, much of traditional eye care is based on a series of unproven assumptions, many of which are wrong. The problem is that prescribing "corrective" lenses is so lucrative that most traditional eye doctors have no desire to change the status quo.

BEHAVIORAL OPTOMETRY

Fortunately for the public, about three thousand behavioral optometrists offer alternative methods of treatment such as vision therapy. We therefore advise you to use the AVI Program under the care of a behavioral optometrist. Look in the Yellow Pages for an optometrist who offers vision therapy or contact one of the following organizations for a referral:

College of Optometrists in Vision Development
353 "H" Street #C, Chula Vista, CA 92010

Optometric Extension Program Foundation
1921 E. Carnegie Avenue #3L, Santa Ana, CA 92705

If you can't find a behavioral optometrist in your area, a traditional eye doctor can provide you with weaker lenses. Remember that many traditional eye doctors feel threatened by vision therapy so don't accept an optometrist or ophthalmologist who tries to discourage you, even if you've been a patient for many years. *The bottom line is that if your vision has gotten worse under his care, his treatment isn't working and you should try something else.* So shop around until you find an eye doctor who is willing to help you achieve your goals.

RESHAPING THE CORNEA

Three major procedures are now available for reshaping the cornea: RK surgery, PRK surgery, and Orthokeratology. These procedures can eliminate or significantly reduce large amounts of myopia and astigmatism. With RK surgery, a scalpel is used to make radial incisions that weaken the cornea and cause it to collapse, thereby changing its curvature. A similar effect is produced with PRK surgery, except that a laser is used to vaporize the cells.

More than a million Americans have undergone RK or PRK surgery. Both operations have a high success rate and most patients become free from "corrective" lenses or significantly reduce their dependency on them. Unfortunately, the cornea suffers major structural damage with RK surgery, and its curvature continues to change for many years, often leading to premature loss of near vision so that reading glasses are needed. PRK surgery appears to be free from these complications and is considered to be safer.

In the hands of a good surgeon the benefits probably outweigh the risks, although only the symptoms are treated, not the underlying cause. Hence in some cases, the myopia continues to increase. All new procedures take many years to become perfected and we're cautiously optimistic that, as surgeons gain more experience, the results will become more consistent, especially if the surgery is followed by vision therapy to make the eyes work more efficiently.

Orthokeratology (Ortho-K) involves wearing special contact lenses that have a better curvature than the cornea. The cornea then adapts to the contact lens by changing its shape. By modifying the shape of the cornea through a series of contact lenses, most people return to normal or near-normal vision within a year. The concept is like using dental braces to straighten teeth.

Although the results are similar to those obtained from surgery, Ortho-K is safer and more reliable because the cornea is not weakened. To maintain the results, it's usually necessary to wear part-time "retainer" lenses. In many cases, these can be inserted at bedtime and removed the next morning, providing natural vision throughout the day.

TIME TO CHANGE THE STATUS QUO

By now it should be abundantly clear that "corrective" lenses often do more harm than good and that major changes are needed in the quality of eye care offered to the public. Although behavioral optometrists can lead by example, they can't force traditional eye doctors to follow. Neither can they compete with the massive TV and Yellow Pages advertising campaigns used to promote these products.

The fact is that the traditional method of prescribing "corrective" lenses has damaged the eyes of tens of millions of people and is a public health problem of major dimensions. The only way to change the status quo is for informed citizens to speak out and spread the word. We can't do it alone. We need your help. If enough people know the truth, it can't be suppressed. If enough people voice their concerns, the eye care establishment will be forced to provide better methods of treatment.

YOU REALLY CAN MAKE A DIFFERENCE

Please tell your family, friends and co-workers. Better still, give them their own copy of the AVI Program. They will thank you for it and you'll have the satisfaction of knowing that you've done something significant to make the world a better place. If you own a business, give the AVI Program to your computer operators and employees who wear glasses, because the stress reduction techniques will help them work more productively. We also encourage health care professionals to give the AVI Program to their patients. By providing a new health care benefit, you will win their gratitude and loyalty.

Contact your local newspaper, TV station, church, school, and PTA association. Many parents and teachers need to know about developmental visual problems and how to stop children from going through life handicapped by inferior vision.

Finally, make sure you actually do the therapy and get results. It's a good idea to join forces with friends once or twice a week for a group therapy session. Even if you don't reach the point where you can throw away your glasses, preventing your vision from getting worse is a lot better than sliding downhill into stronger prescriptions. Thank you for using the AVI Program. Please feel free to contact us if you need any special help or advice.

MAIL THE RESPONSE FORM TODAY

We'd like to hear from you. We want to know about the results you get from the AVI Program and any suggestions for improving future editions. We also provide supporting materials including cassette tapes and special eyecharts for faster results. Just mail the Response Form at the back of the book. You'll receive additional information and a telephone number in case you want to speak to a qualified vision therapist. If the Response Form is missing, write or call:

American Vision Institute
1111 Howe Avenue #235
Sacramento, CA 95825
Tel: (916) 929-8831

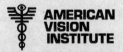
AMERICAN
VISION
INSTITUTE

Appendix

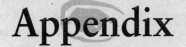

TECHNICAL GUIDE TO PRESCRIBING

LIMITS OF APPLICATION

The AVI Program provides health-conscious individuals with an alternative method of treating common visual problems such as amblyopia, asthenopia, astigmatism, hyperopia, myopia, and presbyopia. The AVI Program may also improve the results obtained from optometric visual training, Ortho-K, and RK and PRK surgery. Therapeutic guidelines are provided for patients with cataract and macular degeneration. Most patients fall into one of the following three categories and should be treated accordingly:

- *Category 1:* Patients with incipient or minor visual problems, such as asthenopia in emmetropia, low myopia, low hyperopia, low astigmatism, or early presbyopia, can often avoid, delay, or eliminate the need for "corrective" lenses. Good results are usually obtained within a month. Asthenopia caused by reading or computer work is particularly easy to treat and most patients report a major reduction in discomfort within a few days.

- *Category 2:* Patients with unstable visual problems, including medium to high astigmatism, hyperopia, myopia, or presbyopia, can often prevent or delay further deterioration and avoid the need for a stronger prescription. Stabilization is usually achieved within a few weeks.

- *Category 3:* Patients with stable visual problems, including medium to high astigmatism, hyperopia, myopia, or presbyopia, can often adapt to a series of undercompensations and reduce their dependency on glasses or contact lenses. Several months of therapy are usually needed to obtain maximum results.

THERAPEUTIC LENS PRESCRIBING

Mydriatic or cycloplegic examinations should be done after functional testing because these drugs increase spherical and chromatic aberrations, complicate retinoscopy, and prevent evaluation of accommodation and accommodative-convergence function. Therapeutic lenses should be prescribed as follows:

- *Category 1:* Patients with incipient visual problems should not be compensated for refractive error. Patients with minor visual problems should receive an undercompensation that gives 20/40 monocular acuity at the distance for which the lenses are normally used. Don't prescribe prism unless absolutely necessary. Ignore low astigmatism up to 1.00D depending on the axis.

- *Category 2:* Since the goal is to stabilize vision through the current prescription, additional lenses are usually not required.

- *Category 3:* Undercompensate to 20/40 monocular acuity at the distance for which the lenses are normally used. Myopes should receive a 20/40 undercompensation for driving. Myopes who engage in long periods of close work should receive a separate prescription that undercompensates them to 20/40 at the working distance. Hyperopes and presbyopes should be undercompensated for close work. Ignore low astigmatism up to 1.00D depending on the axis. Undercompensate larger amounts by one-third. If bifocals are needed, undercompensate both segments.

Continue to periodically reduce the strength of the lenses until the patient achieves the maximum amount of improvement possible. This technique is known as *progressive undercorrection* and is the preferred method of lens prescribing for the AVI Program. The following prescribing techniques may also be helpful in some cases.

STRESS-RELIEVING LENSES

Patients with asthenopia or incipient myopia who engage in long periods of close work should receive *stress-relieving* lenses to prevent accommodation. These lenses should contain the maximum amount of plus acceptable at the working distance. Stress-relieving lenses enable the eyes to perform the nearpoint task as if they were looking at a distant object. Many behavioral optometrists prescribe +0.50D lenses. Although these lenses reduce physiological stress, they don't completely prevent accommodation, and it may be better use more plus power, depending on the patient's ability to accept it. It may also be helpful to prescribe glasses for TV viewing with the maximum amount of plus that will provide satisfactory acuity at a distance of 10 feet. The goal of these lenses is not stress reduction but plus acceptance to reduce accommodation and esophoria.

YOUNG'S FORMULA

The following bifocal prescription will halt or drastically reduce myopic progression and is especially useful for schoolchildren who may not be able to follow a course of vision therapy. The upper lens is for distance vision and is undercompensated by 0.50D; the lower segment is for reading and is +2.00D more than the upper lens. For example, a −4.00D myope will receive a −3.50D upper lens together with a −1.50D lower segment; a −1.25D myope will receive a −0.75D upper lens together with a +1.25 lower segment.

The position of the lower segment is important. The upper edge must reach the lower edge of the pupil under normal lighting conditions with the eyes looking directly ahead. The patient should be instructed to use the lower segment for all reading and close work. Studies with the lower segment below this level enabled the patient to read through the upper segment and the bifocals did not produce such good results.

PATIENT MANAGEMENT

You should meet with patients at regular intervals for lens changes and guidance. We also recommend that you organize weekly seminars of patients with similar visual problems, for example a myopia support group or a presbyopia support group. These can be very rewarding because they allow you to maintain personal contact with large numbers of patients, who appreciate the extra care and attention.

Patients should receive their own copy of the AVI Program, which is protected by international copyright laws and must not be photocopied. If you would like to receive referrals and professional discounts, please mail the Response Form at the end of the book.

ACUITY ENHANCEMENT MECHANISMS

At least seven different mechanisms are responsible for the improvements in acuity obtained by the AVI Program. These mechanisms can operate synergistically and often lead to substantial increases in acuity, which may or may not be accompanied by changes in refractive error.

PERCEPTUAL ENHANCEMENT

Surprisingly, visual acuity is not contingent upon a precise conjugate focus. Even in emmetropia, spherical and chromatic aberrations together with scattering of light by the rods and cones prevent the formation of a perfectly clear retinal image. For this reason, the minimum angle of resolution of the retinal image in normal or "corrected" eyes is about 30 seconds of arc. On the other hand, the minimum angle of resolution of the perceived image is about 5 seconds of arc. In other words, what we actually see is about six times clearer than the retinal image.

This phenomenon is known as *hyperacuity* and means that the brain enhances the signal-to-noise ratio of the retinal data. Computer simulations suggest that the image-processing functions responsible for hyperacuity require a large amount of the visual cortex's computing power.

It follows that stress or sensory overload will decrease the amount of cortical computing power available for image processing and hyperacuity. For the same reason, reducing stress and sensory overload will improve image processing and increase hyperacuity, regardless of the person's age or visual problem. Therapy techniques are Slow Blinking, Blur Zoning, Acuity Chart, Light Therapy, and Palming.

REDUCTION OF THE IOP

Many myopes and presbyopes have excessive IOP caused by the bulging of the lens against the iris, which seems to restrict the flow of liquid into the anterior chamber and may impede drainage through Schlemm's canal. The underlying factors include lenticular growth due to the aging process, chronic nearpoint accommodation, and dietary imbalances such as excessive sugar consumption, which swells the lenticular fibers.

Young's research suggests that excessive IOP can elongate the eyeball and increase myopia. It follows that reducing nearpoint stress and correcting dietary imbalances may reduce IOP and modify the shape and refractive status of the lens and eyeball. Therapy techniques are Light Therapy, Hydrotherapy, and Acupressure.

FORMATION OF A TRANSIENT CONTACT LENS COMPOSED OF TEAR FLUID

Clinical observations have shown that stimulating the blinking mechanism can cover the cornea with a copius amount of tear fluid, which may form a contact lens owing to the meniscus curvature at the eyelids, thereby changing the refractive status of the cornea. Therapy techniques are Fast Blinking, Slow Blinking, and Squeeze Blinking.

EXTENSION OF THE ACCOMMODATIVE AMPLITUDE

With normal use, the ciliary muscle does not expand or contract to its maximum limits. It follows that exercising the ciliary muscle will increase the accommodative amplitude, extend the nearpoint and farpoint, and change the refractive status of the lens. Therapy techniques are Pumping, Tromboning, Acuity Chart, Blur Zoning, and Blur Reading.

MODIFICATION OF THE CILIARY MUSCLE TONICITY

Ciliary muscle tonicity determines the resting state of the lens in the absence of visual stimulation. Modifying the tonicity changes the resting state of the lens and accommodative hysteresis, also modifying the nearpoint and farpoint and changing the refractive status of the lens. Therapy techniques are Pumping, Tromboning, Acuity Chart, Blur Zoning, and Blur Reading.

MODIFICATION OF THE EXTRAOCULAR MUSCLE TONICITY

It is a well known clinical observation that astigmatism can spontaneously change its magnitude and direction. This phenomenon seems to be caused by imbalances in the force exerted by the extraocular muscles on the eyeball, which may deform it and warp the cornea. It follows that correcting the imbalances will modify the extraocular muscle tonicity and change the shape and refractive status of the eyeball and cornea. Therapy techniques are Clock Rotations and Eye Rolls.

REDUCTION OF FIXATION DISPARITY

A blurred image cannot be precisely fixated and leads to convergence errors and diplopia. Since the gross action of the ciliary muscle is determined by convergence, disparity between the spatial location of the object and the point of regard may cause additional loss of focus. It follows that improving extraocular muscle coordination will refine convergence and reduce fixation disparity and diplopia, enabling the eyes to focus more accurately. Therapy techniques are Scanning Chart, Acuity Chart, Nose Fusion, Fusion Chart, and Fusion Pumping.

DOCTRINE OF INFORMED CONSENT

According to Harris and Dister:

It is the patient's right to refuse or consent to a proposed procedure and the doctor's duty to provide sufficient information so that the patient can make the decision in an intelligent, knowledgeable manner. When does this doctrine apply to the optometrist? Nearly all the time. Optometrists cannot rely on existing professional standards as a shield against liability for negligence and must thoroughly advise the patient of potential risks.

Some general rules have evolved. The courts at various times have determined that a health-care practitioner must discuss the following items before a patient can give a valid informed consent: diagnosis, nature, and purpose of treatment; benefits, risks, consequences, and side effects; feasible alternative treatments; probabilities of success; prognosis in the absence of treatment. (JAOA, 58: 230–236, 3/87)

Obviously, the doctrine of informed consent poses serious legal problems for eye doctors who fail to inform their patients that no clinical studies have demonstrated the long-term safety or effectiveness of "corrective" lenses. However, by prescribing a copy of the AVI Program for each patient, conscientious practitioners can conveniently minimize their legal liability by helping their patients learn the truth about these products and alternative methods of treatment.

01•PROFITS YES WEEKEND CULTURE DUKE RESOLVE PENDANT VIRGIN CONCERT OLYMPIC FLAVOR PAGEANT REVELRY POETRY FORGIVE EMPEROR MOZART CLARIFY
02•SCHOLAR KINDRED CHERUB MILLION DIPLOMA SUPRISE VIOLIN DECORUM RAINBOW REVERE QUEEN SAVVY IMAGINE MASSAGE
03•SAVIOR NOTABLE FORTUNE REPLETE AMERICA BIG PRODUCE BANQUET EUROPE TEMPLE SUMMER SETTLE
04•VENTURE EXPRESS LEISURE MONARCH JACKPOT SURPLUS SAVINGS BECAUSE NATURAL
05•RECEIVE BOUNTY DONATE WONDER LIBRARY LETTER STRONG FREEDOM ZOOM
06•HARVEST REGULAR CONQUER ENTRUST TRIUMPH QUALITY ENDORSE
07•RAPIDLY AMUSING INSPIRE THEATER RAPPORT AMIABLE BINGO
08•TWINKLE PRIVACY LAGOON VILLA ESTATE THERAPY HUG
09•GENUINE COMMAND PEACH SHOW COMFORT FOND
10•DIGNITY PARTNER THRIFT HARMONY PEARL FIT
11•ESTATE DEGREE ANTIQUE MANSION HUMOR
12•DEVELOP PRETTY CAVIAR PUPPY EXPLAIN
13•PERFUME ZOO CORDIAL RESPECT FAIR
14•PALACE HOLIDAY SHINE SNUGGLE
15•EMERALD PROTECT TOUCH HOLD
16•COMFORT RAPTURE TRUST JOY
17•ACTION MUSK CONFIDE HUGE
18•ETERNAL ADMIRE EMPATHY
19•BALLET SINCERE BED GIVE
20•REMEDY PURIFY SURVIVE
21•INSIGHT FUNDING VOW
22•EDUCATE HONEY GOLD
23•EXCITE BOLD PROVIDE
24•AWARD EXTRA REGAL
25•AMIABLE BELLE SUN
26•LISTEN GET SECURE
27•LOVE PEACE LORD
28•HEAVEN OVATION
29•NURSE WEALTHY
30•SERENE FLOWER
31•LOVING FAMILY
32•WORSHIP CHIC

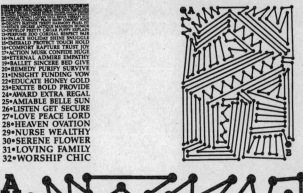

1•SILVER EMBRACE TREASURE SCHOOL WELFARE GENTLE
2•REVOLVE PERFECT CROWN VILLA JEWEL THREAT RUG
3•GENUINE COMMAND PEACH SHOW COMFORT BOND
9•DIGNITY PARTNER THRIFT HARMONY PEARL FIT
11•ESTATE DEGREE ANTIQUE MANSION HUMOR
12•DEVELOP PRETTY CAVIAR PUPPY EXPLAIN
13•PERFUME ZOO CORDIAL RESPECT FAIR
14•PALACE HOLIDAY SHINE SNUGGLE
15•EMERALD PROTECT TOUCH HOLD
16•COMFORT RAPTURE TRUST JOY
17•ACTION MUSK CONFIDE HUGE
18•ETERNAL ADMIRE EMPATHY
19•BALLET SINCERE BED GIVE
20•REMEDY PURIFY SURVIVE
21•INSIGHT FUNDING VOW
22•EDUCATE HONEY GOLD
23•EXCITE BOLD PROVIDE
24•AWARD EXTRA REGAL
25•AMIABLE BELLE SUN
26•LISTEN GET SECURE
27•LOVE PEACE LORD
28•HEAVEN OVATION
29•NURSE WEALTHY
30•SERENE FLOWER
31•LOVING FAMILY
32•WORSHIP CHIC

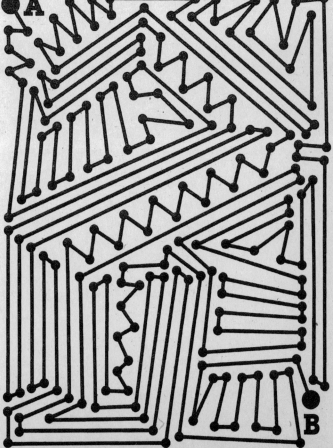

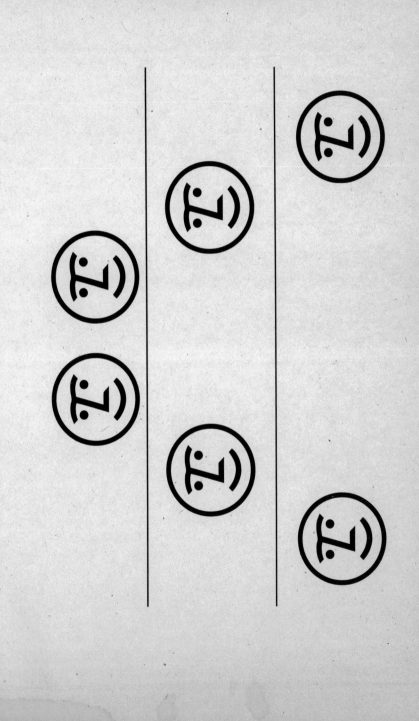

CAR DASHBOARD

REPEAT YOUR
AFFIRMATION
AND PRACTICE
YOUR NEW VISUAL
HABITS AT EVERY
TRAFFIC LIGHT

PUMP

BLINK

BLUR
ZONE

OBEY THE SPEED LAWS
DON'T DRINK AND DRIVE

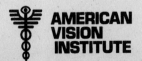

BOOKMARK

STOP!

BEFORE PROCEEDING, TAKE A
DEEP BREATH, REPEAT YOUR
AFFIRMATION, AND PRACTICE
YOUR NEW VISUAL HABITS

PUMP

BLINK

BLUR
ZONE

NOW PUT THE BOOKMARK
ONE PAGE AHEAD AND
CONTINUE READING

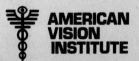

RESPONSE FORM

American Vision Institute
1111 Howe Avenue #235
Sacramento, CA 95825
(916) 929-8831

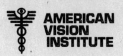
AMERICAN VISION INSTITUTE

Name _____

Address _____

City _____ State _____ Zip _____

Phone: _____ Daytime ( ) Evening ( )

Please describe your visual problem: Astigmatism ( )
Amblyopia ( )   Cataract ( )   Dry Eyes ( )   Eyestrain ( )
Glaucoma ( )   Hyperopia ( )   Macular Degeneration ( )
Myopia ( )   Presbyopia ( )   Strabismus ( )   Other ____

How bad is your visual problem: Minor ( )   Moderate ( )
Major ( )   Stable ( )   Deteriorating ( )   Bifocals ( )   Trifocals ( )

How long have you worn glasses/contacts: _____ yrs

What products and/or services are you interested in:
Audio Tapes ( )   Video Tapes ( )   CD-ROM ( )   Eyecharts ( )
Advanced Therapy Materials ( )   Personal Consultations ( )
Referral to Behavioral Optometrist ( )   Research Listing ( )
Seminars ( )   Vision Enhancing Nutritional Supplements ( )

Would you like us to send information to friends and/or relatives:

Name _____

Address _____

City _____ State _____ Zip _____

over . . .

Name _____

Address _____

City _____ State _____ Zip _____

Name _____

Address _____

City _____ State _____ Zip _____

Name _____

Address _____

City _____ State _____ Zip _____

Name _____

Address _____

City _____ State _____ Zip _____

Name _____

Address _____

City _____ State _____ Zip _____

Name _____

Address _____

City _____ State _____ Zip _____

Name _____

Address _____

City _____ State _____ Zip _____

INDEX